RESTAURANT SURVIVAL GUIDE

1,000+ HEALTHY MENU ITEMS FROM 100 OF THE MOST POPULAR U.S. RESTAURANTS

NICO CHAVANDO

Restaurants reserve the right to change their menus at any time.

Please note that *Restaurant Survival Guide* does not constitute medical advice, and you should consult with your healthcare professional before making any changes to your diet.

ISBN-13: 978-1-7329251-9-9

Restaurants by Cuisine

Asian
Benihana
Panda Express
Pei Wei Asian
Diner
P.F. Chang's
Poke (General)

Mexican
Chili's Grill &
Bar
Chipotle
Chuy's
El Pollo Loco
On The Border
Pollo Tropical
Taco Bell
Taco Cabana
Taco John's

Italian
California Pizza
Kitchen
Carraba's Italian
Grill
Cicis Pizza
Domino's
Jet's Pizza
Maggiano's
Little Italy
Olive Garden
Papa John's

Restaurants by Menu Item

Bowls
BJ's Restaurant & Brewhouse
Bob Evans (fish)
California Pizza Kitchen
Chipotle
El Pollo Loco
First Watch
Jamba Juice
Moe's Southwest Grill
Olive Garden
On the Border Mexican Grill &
Cantina
P.F. Chang's
Pollo Tropical
Qdoba
Taco Bell
Taco Cabana
Tropical Smoothie Café
Yard House
Zoës

Eggs
Bob Evans
Chick-fil-A
Corner Bakery Cafe
Cracker Barrel Old Country
Store
Denny's
First Watch
IHOP
O'Charley's
Panera Bread

Eggs (cont.)
Perkins Restaurant & Bakery
Taco Cabana
Taco John's
The Cheesecake Factory
Village Inn
Waffle House

Grilled Chicken Sandwiches
Bar Louie
Burger King
Carl's Jr.
Carraba's Italian Grill
Cheddar's Scratch Kitchen
Corner Bakery Cafe
Cracker Barrel Old Country Store
Culver's
Dairy Queen
Dave and Buster's
Denny's
Firehouse Subs
Freddy's Frozen Custard and Steakburgers
Hardee's
Hungry Howie's
Longhorn Steakhouse
McDonald's
Ruby Tuesday
Steak 'n Shake

Pasta
Maggiano's
Olive Garden

Pizza
Bertucci's

Poke
P.F. Chang's
Poke (General)
Yard House

Smoothies
Jamba Juice
Tropical Smoothie Café

Tacos
Chuy's
El Pollo Loco
Moe's Southwest Grill
On The Border Mexican Grill & Cantina
Qdoba
Red Lobster (fish & chicken)
Taco Cabana
Taco John's
The Cheesecake Factory

Table of Contents

About the Author

Nico Chavando is the founder of Ocinator.com and the Ocinator Fitness Program. He obtained his Product Design Degree from Stanford University. There, he experimented with different approaches to being fit and healthy long-term.

Nico used his background in Design Thinking to identify a problem affecting 40% of the population, obesity and obesity-related diseases, and to offer an attainable, easy solution. While trendy diets and workout programs grow in popularity, the obesity rate is not decreasing. In fact, obesity-related conditions like heart disease, stroke, type 2 diabetes, and certain types of cancer continue to be some of the leading causes of preventable premature death.

Nico found that many current diets make people think that eating healthily involves counting calories, limiting food consumption, complicated meal preparation, avoiding good protein sources, and/or eliminating carbs. Unfortunately, these common misconceptions about healthy eating lead some to adopt unrealistic and possibly harmful diets. These painful diets rely on dramatic changes of habits and often cause constant feelings of hunger, decreased mental sharpness, and negative changes in mood including crankiness, hostility, and depression.

1 in 3 Americans eats out on any given day, either for work or social reasons, because we are busy, do not like to cook, or just because we prefer eating out! Many of us are concerned with our weight and overall health and would like to eat healthy foods at restaurants, but end up ordering unhealthy menu items. This is because we either do not know how to modify restaurant orders to make them

healthy, or because tweaking orders is a hassle to think about when we are in a rush.

Helping restaurant-goers eat a sound meal is a need that was largely unmet by diet books… until now.

We need a quick and easy guide to help us eat in a healthy way and feel good without becoming chefs. So, Nico created *Restaurant Survival Guide*. With over 1,000 healthy menu options, this book helps busy folks like you to eat on the go, healthily, and without the pain that many other diets produce. It is an ongoing solution to promote long-term health.

Restaurant Survival Guide has helped many people of all ages eat healthily every day and be amazed at the results. You can have the strength, energy, and positivity provided by delicious, healthy food and be fit! Nico hopes this guide will help you and many more feel great long-term too.

Introduction

Busy and want something quick to eat? Don't like to cook? Traveling? Or just love eating out? *Restaurant Survival Guide* was designed to show you exactly how to choose healthy menu options at the most popular chain restaurants in the U.S.

Learn how to eat healthily without starving yourself or counting calories!

The latest medical research shows that "a calorie is not a calorie," meaning that in a healthy lifestyle the quality of the food eaten matters more than the quantity of food eaten. Common sense tells us that it is healthier to eat 100 calories of vegetables than 100 calories of chocolate cake.

Restaurant Survival Guide lists healthy food you can eat at restaurants to help you lose weight the simple way, without the pain of starvation of no-carb diets.

The following pages help explain how *Restaurant Survival Guide* is effective and why you will benefit from the following suggestions.

<u>Keys to Remember</u>

1. Small changes make a huge difference.
2. Be brave.
3. Be consistent.
4. Think results and after-effects… to say no to junk food now.

1. Small changes make a huge difference.

It might seem like the difference between white bread and whole grain bread, water and lemonade, dressing and no dressing, are of little significance. False. These small changes are what allow you to lose fat without spending all day doing cardio.

Know that the small changes you make add up and help sculpt an amazing body through a realistic and physically painless process. Our good small choices add up for the better!

2. Be brave.

Do not be afraid to ask servers to modify menu options! You are paying for the food which directly affects how healthy you look and feel. Be brave and ask for the food you need to succeed.

3. Be consistent.

Do not take days off. Of course, at first it may be difficult to give up certain things like white bread, dressing, cheese, sugary foods, and butter. Ease off these foods, and notice how your taste buds improve and how great you look and feel.

4. Think results and after-effects... to say no to junk food now.

When resisting the temptation to eat unhealthy food, think about how unhealthy junk food makes you feel after you eat it. The healthier you eat, the more you will be able to notice how badly junk food makes the body feel. Thinking about how badly junk food makes your body feel can help stop you from eating junk food in the first place.

<u>General Healthy Food Guidelines</u>

Stay away from refined grains.

The prominent advice in medicine today indicates how to

lose weight in a healthy way: stay away from products with *refined grain* and products with added sugar. Also, eat lots of vegetables. The key: *refined grain* carbs are bad. On the other hand, *whole grain* carbs are good.

Refined grain carbs are unhealthy because they have been stripped of the nutrients that whole grains have. But because *whole grain* carbs have those nutrients, they are good for you.

Studies have shown that not eating whole grain carbs could lead to: poorer memory-based task performance, bad breath, and increased anger, depression, anxiety, irritability, and hostility.

On the other hand, eating whole grain carbs could lead to positive effects by allowing the soluble fiber, found in whole grain carbs, to:

- Decrease LDL (bad) cholesterol
- Increase good HDL cholesterol
- Increase dietary fiber
- Help promote fat loss
- Prevent fat gain
- Lower the risk of diabetes

Refined grains do not provide these potential benefits.

Stay away from products with added sugar and artificial sweeteners.

The more you stay away from products with added sugar, the sweeter naturally sweet food, like fruit, will taste!

Stay away from: soda, most desserts, dressings, syrups, jams, jellies, etc. Instead, try eating naturally sweet food like fruit.

Look out for hidden sugars and additives. For example, dressing contains too much added sugar as well as saturated fat and sodium that can lead to increased body fat and feelings of hunger.

Research changes regarding the side effects of artificial sweeteners, so it is best to avoid them.

Again, small changes like eating fruit and getting rid of salad dressing add up and make a huge difference!

Balance your meats.

Though this book lists beef menu options, it is not a free pass to eat beef during every meal. Try eating mostly chicken and fish. Consuming too much red meat can be unhealthy.

Eat lots of vegetables.

We all know the many benefits of eating most vegetables! Let's have more fiber and freshness.

<u>Overall Fitness</u>

Restaurant Survival Guide is intended to help users lose body fat. To help you sculpt abs and other muscles, we recommend the Ocinator Fitness Program as the ideal companion to this book. Ocinator workouts are simple and do not aim for sweat and exhaustion.

On the contrary, Ocinator workouts were designed to minimize workout time (20 minutes/day) and pain so that users can realistically maintain results and a positive long-term change in fitness lifestyle. See Ocinator.com for more details.

Both *Restaurant Survival Guide* and Ocinator Fitness aim to make obtaining and maintaining long-term fitness results simple and realistic.

Now… it's time to enjoy all your new restaurant menu options <u>and</u> feel great!

General Ordering Guidelines

Be comfortable asking for:

- Whole grains, brown rice - instead of white/refined carbs*
- Food that is steamed, baked/grilled with no/minimal oil
- Lemon slices, vinegar, mustard, guacamole/avocados, or fresh salsa, pepper and other herbs - instead of dressings, condiments and sauces that contain extra oils/fats

*Including free appetizers

General Cuisine Guidelines

Mexican

Stay away from: chips, cheese, Mexican rice, white flour tortillas, and hard-shell (fried) tortillas.

Choose soft corn tortillas or brown rice instead.

Italian

Stay away from: white flour (bread, pizza dough, pasta dough) and cheese.

Choose whole wheat options.

Asian

Stay away from: stir fry (ask for food to be cooked with little to no oil), refined grain (white rice and noodles), butter (on meat, especially), and sauce.

Choose steamed foods, brown rice, and ginger and pepper.

American

Stay away from: fried food, cheese, sauce, dressing/vinaigrette, and white bread/buns (including free appetizers).

Choose grilled and whole wheat options.

*Stick to water or low-fat milk, unless we list drink items like healthy smoothies. (No soda, juice, or alcohol.)

Restaurant Menu Items With Healthy Tweaks

Applebee's

Drink: Water

Appetizers

- House Salad
  without: cheese, croutons, and dressing
- Chicken Tortilla Soup
  without: tortilla strips and cheese
- Tomato Basil
  without: croutons and cheese

Sides/Extras

- Baked Potato
  without: butter, sour cream, cheese, bacon, etc.
- Steamed Broccoli

Steaks & Ribs

- 6 oz. or 8 oz. Top Sirloin
  without: butter. see above for sides/extras

Chicken

- Cedar Grilled Lemon Chicken
  without: cranberry-pecan rice (quinoa instead) and vinaigrette/dressing (ask for lemon slices instead)

Salads

instead of dressing, ask for: lemon, pepper, vinegar, guacamole/avocados, or fresh salsa

- Southwest Steak Salad
  without: chimichurri, cheese, tortilla strips, and ranch
- Grilled Chicken Salad
  without: cheese and dressing

Seafood

- Cedar Salmon
  without: maple mustard glaze. see above for sides/extras

Applebee's (2)

Drink: Water

Sandwiches

- Clubhouse Grille
  without: potato bread (instead, whole wheat/grain bread or lettuce bun)
  without: bacon, cheese, honey bbq, mayo, and fries

Burgers

Classic Burger
without: white bread bun (instead, whole wheat/grain bread or lettuce bun), cheese, sauce, pickles, and fries

Arby's

Drink: Water

Entrée

- Turkey Avocado Club
  without: honey wheat bread (lettuce bun instead), bacon, and mayo
- Roast Turkey Farmhouse Salad
  without: honey wheat bread, bacon, and cheese
- Roast Turkey Wrap
  without: white flour wrap (wheat grain wrap instead), bacon, cheese, mayonnaise, and ranch

Sides

- Chopped Side Salad
  without: cheese, croutons, and dressing

Au Bon Pain

Drink: Water

Soups

- 12 Veggie
- Vegetable Beef & Barley

Sandwiches

- Turkey Sandwich
  without: Swiss cheese and honey pecan spread
- Black Angus Roast Beef Sandwich
  without: cheddar and dijonnaise

Wraps

- Napa Chicken With Avocado
  without: white flour wrap (whole wheat wrap instead), aïoli, and lemon shallot vinaigrette
- Harvest Turkey
  without: mayo and cheddar

Salads

instead of dressing, ask for: lemon, pepper, vinegar, guacamole/avocados, or fresh salsa

- Chicken Cobb with Avocado
  without: bacon
- Vegetarian Deluxe
- Harvest Turkey
  without: goat cheese

Bar Louie

Drink: Water

Sandwiches

- California Chicken Club
  without: bacon, pepper jack, and ranch. with side of fruit or salad without dressing, cheese, and croutons

Burgers

- Ask for a burger on whole grain bread with just the beef patty, tomato, and lettuce (without cheese, sauce, etc.)

Benihana

Drink: Water

Entrées

- Hibachi Chicken
  without: butter on chicken and vegetables
- Hibachi Shrimp
  without: butter on shrimp and vegetables
- Filet Mignon
  without: butter on filet mignon and vegetables
- Hibachi Steak
  without: butter on steak and vegetables
- Beef Julienne
  without: butter on beef and vegetables

Sides

- Benihana Salad
  without: dressing. with vinegar instead
- Brown Rice
- Miso Soup

Bertucci's

Drink: Water

Brick Oven Pizzas

Multigrain Dough

+ *sliced cherry peppers, broccoli, mushrooms, bell peppers, onions, diced plum tomatoes, sliced tomatoes, spinach, and/or arugula*

+ (optional) *roasted garlic, roasted black olives, roasted zucchini, roasted peppers, roasted artichokes, roasted eggplant, and/or roasted button mushrooms*

+ (optional) *red wine vinegar*

+ (optional) *chicken, meatballs, and/or rosemary ham*

without: cheese, bacon, pepperoni, sauce, and dressing

Pasta Classics

- Spaghetti & Polpette (Meatballs)
  without: white flour pasta (whole wheat linguine instead) and cheese
- Chicken Domani (with Grilled Chicken substitute)
  without: white flour pasta (whole wheat linguine instead), cheese, and white wine sauce (pomodoro instead)
- Rigatoni, Broccoli, and Chicken (with Grilled Chicken substitute)
  without: white flour pasta (whole wheat linguine instead), cheese, sautéed breaded chicken (grilled chicken instead), white wine sauce (pomodoro instead)
- Rigatoni, Broccoli, and Shrimp (with Grilled Shrimp)
  without: white flour pasta (whole wheat linguine instead), cheese, and white wine or lemon-garlic cream sauce (pomodoro instead)

Soups

- Minestrone
  without: cheese
- Lentil Soup
  without: caramelized onions, sautéed garlic, evoo, balsamic vinegar, and hand-chopped parsley

Bertucci's (2)

Drink: Water

Starters

- Polpette (Meatballs)
  without: cheese
- Antipasto
  without: mozzarella, balsamic fig drizzle, pecorino romano, salami, stuffed green olives with grilled prosciutto rolled around fresh mozzarella, and grilled rosemary focaccia

Salads

instead of dressing, ask for: lemon, pepper, vinegar, guacamole/avocados, or fresh salsa

- Farmhouse Salad (with Grilled Shrimp, Grilled Chicken, or Grilled Salmon)
  without: cheese, pepperoni, balsamic fig glaze, and vinaigrette/dressing
- Shrimp & Spinach Gorgonzola Salad (with Grilled Shrimp, Grilled Chicken, or Grilled Salmon)
  without: cheese and vinaigrette/dressing
- Insalata
  without: cheese and vinaigrette/dressing
- Shrimp Mediterraneo Salad (with Grilled Shrimp, Grilled Chicken, or Grilled Salmon)
  without: cheese and vinaigrette/dressing
- Grilled Chicken Caesar Salad
  without: cheese, croutons, and vinaigrette/dressing
- Baby Arugula & Grilled Chicken
  without: vinaigrette/dressing

Specialty Entrées

- Bistecca
  without: sautéed spinach (grilled instead) and Marsala sauce (pomodoro instead)
- Roasted Eggplant Pomodoro
  without: spaghetti (whole grain linguine instead) and mozzarella

Bertucci's (3)

Drink: Water

<u>Seafood Entrées</u>

- Salmon
  without: sautéed spinach (grilled or cooked with little to no oil instead). ask for potatoes to be grilled or cooked without oil
- Cod Limone
  without: cheese and angel hair pasta (whole wheat linguine instead)

<u>Chicken Entrées</u>

- Chicken Piccata
  without: sautéed breaded chicken (grilled chicken instead), egg fettuccine (whole wheat linguine instead), white wine sauce (pomodoro instead), and cheese
- Chicken Anna Maria
  without: sautéed breaded chicken (grilled chicken instead), egg fettuccine (whole wheat linguine instead), and cream sauce (pomodoro instead)
- Chicken Marsala
  without: Marsala wine sauce (pomodoro instead), spaghetti (whole wheat linguine instead), and cheese. ask for potatoes to be cooked with little to no oil

Remember:
Small changes make a huge difference.
Know that the small changes you make add up and help sculpt an amazing body through a realistic and physically painless process. Our small choices add up for the better!

BJ's Restaurant & Brewhouse

Drink: Water

Entrées

- Enlightened Chicken Quinoa Bowl
  ask for steamed, not sautéed, vegetables and very little olive oil
- Enlightened Lemon Thyme Chicken
  ask for steamed, not sautéed, vegetables
  without lemon thyme sauce
- Enlightened Fire-Roasted Barbacoa Chicken
  without: feta cheese and crema
- House Top Sirloin
  with two of the following sides: asparagus (steamed), black beans, bowl of soup, salad (no cheese and dressing), broccoli (steamed), quinoa
- BJ's Classic Rib-Eye
  with two of the following sides: asparagus (steamed), black beans, bowl of soup, salad (no cheese and dressing), broccoli (steamed), quinoa

Soups

- Chicken Tortilla Soup
  without: tortilla strips (usually fried). ask for soft corn tortillas instead, if available
- Tomato Bisque
  without croutons

Salads

instead of dressing, ask for: lemon, pepper, vinegar, guacamole/avocados, or fresh salsa

- House Salad
  without: Parmesan cheese and croutons

Bob Evans

Drink: Water

Entrées

- Grilled Chicken Breast
  without white bread. see below for sides
- Grilled Salmon
  without white bread. see below for sides
- USDA Choice Sirloin
  without white bread. see below for sides
- Handcrafted Deli Turkey Sandwich
  without: marble wheat bread (whole wheat/grain bread or lettuce bun instead), Swiss cheese, and mayo. instead of fries, see below for healthy sides

Family Meals

- Grilled Chicken Breasts
  with two of the following sides: asparagus (steamed), black beans, bowl of soup, salad (no cheese and dressing), broccoli (steamed), quinoa

Soups

- Chicken & Noodles
  without: noodles
- Hearty Beef Vegetable Soup

Sides

- Seasonal Fresh Fruit
- Farmhouse Garden Salad
  without: tortilla strips, cheddar cheese, and dressing

Bob Evans (2)

Drink: Water

<u>Breakfast</u>

ask for food to be cooked without butter and with little to no oil

- Rise & Shine
  with ham and fruit (as a side) and more fruit instead of white bread (get whole wheat/grain bread if available) or potatoes cooked with little to no oil
  without: white bread, biscuits, hash browns, fries, and grits
- Sirloin Steak & Farm Fresh Eggs
  with ham and fruit (as a side) and more fruit instead of white bread (get whole wheat/grain bread if available) or potatoes cooked with little to no oil
  without: white bread, biscuits, hash browns, fries, and grits

<u>Salads</u>

instead of dressing, ask for: lemon, pepper, vinegar, guacamole/avocados, or fresh salsa

- Wildfire Chicken Salad
  without: tortilla strips, cheddar cheese, and dressing
- Cranberry Pecan Chicken Salad
  without: bacon, bleu cheese, and dressing
- Cobb Salad
  without: bacon, bleu cheese, and dressing

Remember:
The latest medical research shows that "a calorie is not a calorie," meaning that in a healthy lifestyle the quality of the food eaten matters more than the quantity of food eaten. Common sense tells us that it is healthier to eat 100 calories of vegetables than 100 calories of chocolate cake.

Bonefish Grill

Drink: Water

Dinner

- Chilean Sea Bass
  without: butter or sauce
- Atlantic Salmon
  without: butter or sauce
- Ahi Tuna Steak
  without: butter or sauce
- Rainbow Tuna
  without: butter or sauce
- Filet Mignon
  without: butter
- Bone-In Ribeye Steak
  without: butter
- Sirloin Steak
  without: butter
- Lily's Chicken
  without: goat cheese and lemon basil sauce
- Dynamite-Style Shrimp
  without: aïoli and feta cheese
- Cold Water Lobster Tails
  without: butter

Salads

instead of dressing, ask for: lemon, pepper, vinegar, guacamole/avocados, or fresh salsa

- Bonefish Cobb Salad
  without: blue cheese, bacon, and ranch
- Bonefish House Salad
  without: citrus herb vinaigrette
- Grilled Salmon Superfood Salad
  without: feta, vinaigrette, and citrus aïoli

Boston Market

Drink: Water

Entrées

- Rotisserie Chicken (Half Chicken, Quarter White, or Three-Piece Dark)
  see below for sides
- Rotisserie Turkey Breast
  see below for sides

Soups

- Rotisserie Chicken Soups
  without noodles

Salads

instead of dressing, ask for: lemon, pepper, vinegar, guacamole/avocados, or fresh salsa

- House Salad
  without: Parmesan cheese and croutons

Sides

- Fresh Steamed Vegetables
- Salad
  without: dressing and cheese

Buffalo Wild Wings

Drink: Water

<u>Salads</u>

instead of dressing, ask for: lemon, pepper, vinegar, guacamole/avocados, or fresh salsa

- Santa Fe Salad (Grilled Chicken)
  without: cheese, tortilla strips, ranch, and flour tortillas (instead, get soft corn tortillas if available)
- Garden Chicken Salad (Grilled Chicken)
  without: Parmesan, croutons, vinaigrette, and toast
- Side Salad
  without: Parmesan, croutons, vinaigrette, and toast

<u>Tenders</u>

- Naked Tenders
  without: sauce and fries (ask for a salad without dressing, croutons, and cheese as a substitute for fries)

Burger King

Drink: Water

<u>Sandwiches</u>

- Grilled Chicken Sandwich
  without: white bread bun (instead, lettuce bun or whole wheat bun if available) and mayo
  Why not the potato bun? It contains refined flour, which contributes to weight gain.

<u>Salads</u>

instead of dressing, ask for: lemon, pepper, vinegar, guacamole/avocados, or fresh salsa

- Chicken Garden Salad
  without: croutons, cheese, and dressing/vinaigrette
- Garden Side Salad
  without: croutons, cheese, and dressing/vinaigrette

California Pizza Kitchen

Drink: Water

<u>Soups</u>

- Sedona Tortilla
  without: tortilla strips (unless they are baked, not fried). instead, get soft corn tortillas if available

<u>Power Bowls</u>

- Banh Mi Bowl
  without vinaigrette
- Santa Fe Bowl
  without ranch

<u>Salads</u>

instead of dressing, ask for: lemon, pepper, vinegar, guacamole/avocados, or fresh salsa

- Roasted Veggie (Grilled Chicken or Shrimp)
  without vinaigrette
- Waldorf Chicken
  without: vinaigrette and candied walnuts
- California Cobb
  without: bacon and dressing
- Quinoa + Arugula
  without: feta and vinaigrette

<u>Main Plates</u>

- Hearth-Roasted Halibut
  without creamy farro
- Cedar Plank Salmon
  without feta

Note: Cauliflower pizza dough is unhealthy, as it contains mozzarella cheese

Captain D's Seafood Kitchen

Drink: Water

<u>Salads</u>

instead of dressing, ask for: lemon, pepper, vinegar, guacamole/avocados, or fresh salsa

- Wild Alaskan Salmon Salad
  without: dressing and breadstick

<u>Sides</u>

- Side Salad
  without dressing
- Broccoli
  without feta
- Baked Potato
  without: butter and sour cream
- Corn
  without butter

<u>Grilled Meals</u>

for each of the items below: without white rice (get brown rice if available) and breadstick. ask for one of the sides above as a replacement

- Shrimp Skewers
- Blackened Tilapia
- Wild Alaskan Salmon
- Grilled White Fish and Shrimp Skewer
- Lemon Pepper White Fish

Captain D's Seafood Kitchen (2)

Drink: Water

<u>What's New</u>

- Tilapia & Shrimp Skewer
  without: white rice (get brown rice if available) and breadstick. instead, ask for one of the sides above as a replacement
- Lemon Pepper Steamed Shrimp
  without ketchup or dressing

Carl's Jr.

Drink: Water

<u>Sandwiches</u>

- Low Carb Charbroiled Chicken Club
  without: honey wheat bun (lettuce bun instead), bacon, cheese, and mayo

<u>Salads</u>

instead of dressing, ask for: lemon, pepper, vinegar, guacamole/avocados, or fresh salsa

- Charbroiled Chicken Salad
  without: cheese, croutons, and dressing
- Side Salad
  without: cheese, croutons, and dressing

Carraba's Italian Grill

Drink: Water

Soups

- Minestrone

Salads

instead of dressing, ask for: lemon, pepper, vinegar, guacamole/avocados, or fresh salsa

- Italian Salad
  without vinaigrette/dressing
- Johnny Rocco Salad
  without: vinaigrette/dressing and ricotta
- Italian Side Salad
  without vinaigrette/dressing
- House Side Salad
  without vinaigrette/dressing

Main Plates

order any of the following without butter or sauce
ask for minimal olive oil

- Tuscan-Grilled Sirloin
- Tuscan-Grilled Filet
- Tuscan-Grilled Ribeye
- Tuscan-Grilled Chicken

Seafood

- Tomato Basil Salmon
  ask to be cooked without butter and with little to no oil
- Wood-Grilled Tilapia
  without: balsamic glaze. ask for minimal olive oil
- California Veggie
  without: cheese

Carraba's Italian Grill (2)

Drink: Water

<u>Pasta</u>

- If a whole wheat/grain pasta is available, get it with marinara sauce and meatballs
  without cheese

<u>Sides</u>

- Grilled Asparagus
  without cheese
- Broccoli
  ask for broccoli to be grilled or steamed and cooked with little to no oil

Remember:
Be brave.
Do not be afraid to ask waiters to modify menu options! You are paying for the food which directly affects how healthy you look and feel. Be brave and ask for the food you need to succeed.

Chick-fil-A

Drink: Water

Breakfast

- Egg White Grill
  without cheese
- Sunflower Multigrain Bagel

Salads

instead of dressing, ask for: lemon, pepper, vinegar, guacamole/avocados, or fresh salsa

- Spicy Southwest Salad
  without: cheese, tortilla strips, and dressing
- Market Salad
  without: cheese and dressing

Entrées

- Grilled Chicken Cool Wrap
  without cheese
- Grilled Chicken Sandwich
  without sauce
- Grilled Nuggets
  without sauce

Sides

- Chicken Noodle Soup
  without saltine crackers
- Side Salad
  without cheese
- Superfood Side
  without: vinaigrette/dressing, dried sour cherries, and roasted nuts (if sweetened. if plain, they're ok to eat)
- Fruit Cup

Chili's Grill & Bar

Drink: Water

Sides

- Steamed Broccoli
- Black Beans
  without cheese
- Corn
  without butter
- Grilled Asparagus
  without butter

Salads

instead of dressing, ask for: lemon, pepper, vinegar, guacamole/avocados, or fresh salsa

- Santa Fe Chicken Salad
  without vinaigrette/dressing
- Quesadilla Explosion Salad
  without: ricotta and vinaigrette/dressing
- Grilled Chicken Salad
  without vinaigrette/dressing
- Caribbean Salad with Seared Shrimp or Grilled Chicken
  without vinaigrette/dressing

Tacos

- Grilled Chicken or Steak Tacos
  with: soft corn tortillas, avocado, pico, and cilantro
  without: flour tortillas, cheese, coleslaw, and Mexican rice (instead, ask for steamed broccoli, side salad without dressing, cheese, and croutons, or more beans without cheese)

Chili's Grill & Bar (2)

Drink: Water

<u>Guiltless Grill</u>

- Margarita Grilled Chicken
  without: tortilla strips and Mexican rice (instead, ask for steamed broccoli, side salad without dressing, cheese, and croutons, or beans without cheese)
- Grilled Chicken Salad
  without: cheese and vinaigrette/dressing
- Ancho Salmon
  without: sauce and cheese. more broccoli instead of white rice (or get brown rice, if available)
- 6 oz. Classic Sirloin with Grilled Avocado
  without sauce. and the salad without cheese and dressing

<u>Lunch Specials</u>

- Bacon Avocado Grilled Chicken Sandwich
  without: white bread (whole wheat/grain bread instead), bacon, cheese, sautéed onions (grilled or raw onions instead), mayo, butter, and fries (instead, ask for steamed broccoli, side salad without dressing, cheese, and croutons, or beans without cheese)
- California Turkey Club
  without: white bread (whole wheat/grain bread instead), bacon, cheese, sautéed onions (grilled or raw onions instead), mayo, and fries (instead, ask for steamed broccoli, side salad without dressing, cheese, and croutons, or beans without cheese)
- Chipotle Chicken Fresh Mex Bowl
  without: cheese, tortilla strips, dressing/sauce (salsa is okay), and Mexican rice (instead, ask for steamed broccoli, side salad without dressing, cheese, and croutons, or beans without cheese)

Chili's Grill & Bar (3)

Drink: Water

<u>Fajitas</u>

ask for fajitas to be cooked with little to no oil

- Chicken Fajitas
  without Mexican rice. instead, ask for steamed broccoli, side salad without dressing (lemon instead), cheese, and croutons, or more beans without cheese
- Steak Fajitas
  without Mexican rice. instead, ask for steamed broccoli, side salad without dressing (lemon instead), cheese, and croutons, or more beans without cheese
- Black Bean & Veggie Fajitas
  without Mexican rice. instead, ask for steamed broccoli, side salad without dressing (lemon instead), cheese, and croutons, or more beans without cheese

Remember:

Be consistent.

Do not take days off. Of course, at first it may be difficult to give up certain things like white bread, dressing, cheese, sugary foods, and butter. Ease off these foods, and notice how your taste buds improve and how great you look and feel.

Chipotle Mexican Grill

Drink: Water

<u>Bowl</u>

- Steak
  with: brown rice, black beans, fresh tomato salsa (mild), roasted chili-corn salsa (medium), lettuce, guacamole (guacamole is extra charge)
- Chicken
  with: brown rice, black beans, fresh tomato salsa (mild), roasted chili-corn salsa (medium), lettuce, guacamole (guacamole is extra charge)
- Barbacoa
  with: brown rice, black beans, fresh tomato salsa (mild), roasted chili-corn salsa (medium), lettuce, guacamole (guacamole is extra charge)

<u>Salad</u>

instead of dressing, ask for: lemon, pepper, vinegar, guacamole/avocados, or fresh salsa

- Steak
  with: brown rice, black beans, fresh tomato salsa (mild), roasted chili-corn salsa (medium), lettuce, guacamole (guacamole is extra charge)
- Chicken
- *with: brown rice, black beans, fresh tomato salsa (mild), roasted chili-corn salsa (medium), lettuce, guacamole (guacamole is extra charge)*
- Barbacoa
  with: brown rice, black beans, fresh tomato salsa (mild), roasted chili-corn salsa (medium), lettuce, guacamole (guacamole is extra charge)

Chuck E. Cheese's

Drink: Water

Wraps and Sandwiches

- Club Wrap
  without: white flour tortilla (whole wheat tortilla instead), bacon, cheese, and mayo

Endless Salad Bar

instead of dressing, ask for: lemon, pepper, vinegar, guacamole/avocados, or fresh salsa

- Garden-Fresh Salad Bar
  get any vegetables you want
  without: cheese, dressing, and pasta salad

Start Your Party Right

- Veggie Platter
  without dressing

Remember:

Think results and after-effects... to say no to junk food now.

When resisting the temptation to eat unhealthy food, think about how unhealthy junk food makes you feel after you eat it. The healthier you eat, the more you will be able to notice how badly junk food makes the body feel.

Chuy's

Drink: Water

Appetizers

- Guacamole
  without: chips. ask for soft corn tortillas instead

Salads & Soups

instead of dressing, ask for: lemon, pepper, vinegar, guacamole/avocados, or fresh salsa

- Grilled Chicken Salad
  without: cheese or dressing
- Tortilla Soup
  without cheese and tortilla strips. instead of tortilla strips (usually fried), ask for soft corn tortillas

Tacos

- Soft Tacos (Chicken or Beef)
  ask for soft corn tortillas instead of flour tortillas
  without cheese
- Tacos Al Carbon (Chicken or Beef)
  ask for soft corn tortillas instead of flour tortillas
  without cheese

Fajitas

ask for fajitas to be cooked with little to no oil

- Chicken Fajitas
  without: cheese, sour cream, rice, and flour tortillas. ask for more beans or vegetables instead of rice. ask for soft corn tortillas instead of flour tortillas
- Steak Fajitas
  without: cheese, sour cream, rice, and flour tortillas. ask for more beans or vegetables instead of rice. ask for soft corn tortillas instead of flour tortillas

Cheddar's Scratch Kitchen

Drink: Water

<u>Soups</u>

- Homemade Baked Potato Soup
  without: cheese and bacon
- Tortilla Soup
  without cheese. instead of tortilla strips (usually fried), ask for soft corn tortillas

<u>Salads</u>

instead of dressing, ask for: lemon, pepper, vinegar, guacamole/avocados, or fresh salsa

- Grilled Chicken Pecan Salad
  without: cheese and dressing
- Salmon & Strawberry Salad
  without: cheese and dressing

<u>Sides</u>

- Steamed Fresh Broccoli
- Baked Potato
  without: cream, cheese, butter, bacon etc.
  optional: pepper, chives

<u>Fish</u>

- Grilled Salmon
  without: cheese and dressing
- Grilled White Fish
  without: cheese and dressing

<u>Steak</u>

see above for sides

- 6 or 8 oz. Top Sirloin Steak
- 12 oz. Ribeye
- 20 oz. Bone-In Ribeye

Cheddar's Scratch Kitchen (2)

Drink: Water

Lighter Side

- Lemon Pepper White Fish
  without: salad dressing and white rice (brown rice instead). if brown rice is not available, ask for more beans or salad/vegetables (without dressing, cheese, and croutons) as a substitute
- Grilled Baja Chicken
  without white rice (brown rice instead). if not available, ask for more beans without cheese or salad/vegetables (without dressing, cheese, and croutons) as a substitute

Cicis Pizza

Drink: Water

Soups & Mini Salads

- Salad Mix
  without: cheese and dressing
  with (optional): grape tomatoes, grape tomatoes, baby carrots, sliced radish, green bell peppers, sliced cucumbers, black olives, broccoli florets, sliced red onions, sliced mushrooms, pineapple, jalapeños, banana peppers

Corner Bakery Cafe

Drink: Water

Featured Flavors

- Farmers Scrambler
  without: cheese and white bread (get whole wheat/grain toast)
- Chilled Swiss Oats
  without: raisin pecan sweet crisp

Morning Favorites

- Anaheim Scrambler
  without: bacon, cheese, and white bread (get whole wheat/grain toast)

Oatmeals & Yogurt

- Steel-Cut Oatmeal
  without: brown sugar and sweet crisp
- Berry Almond Swiss Oats
  without sweet crisp

Fresh Salads

instead of dressing, ask for: lemon, pepper, vinegar, guacamole/avocados, or fresh salsa

- Santa Fe Ranch
  without: cheese, tortilla strips, and ranch
- Chopped Salad
  without: bacon, cheese, and dressing/vinaigrette
- Harvest Salad
  without: cheese, pecan sweet crisps, and dressing/vinaigrette

Signature Sandwiches

- D.C. Chicken Salad
  without mayo
- Uptown Turkey Avocado
  without: bacon and mayo

Corner Bakery Cafe (2)

Drink: Water

Soups

- Roasted Tomato Basil Soup

Power Flats

- Avocado and Spinach
  without cheese

Keys to Remember

1. Small changes make a huge difference.
2. Be brave.
3. Be consistent.
4. Think results and after-effects… to say no to junk food now.

Cracker Barrel Old Country Store

Drink: Water

Breakfast

- Good Morning Breakfast
  without: turkey sausage and grits. ask for more fruit or eggs instead
- Custom: ask for scrambled eggs with fruit on the side

Lunch & Dinner

- Southern Chicken Salad
  without: dressing, Parmesan cheese, croutons, deviled eggs, and dressing. ask for hard-boiled eggs instead
- Lemon Pepper Grilled Rainbow Trout Plate
  with sides: fruit, steamed broccoli, carrots, or plain corn
- Grilled Chicken Salad
  without: dressing, cheese, croutons, deviled eggs, crackers, and dressing. ask for hard-boiled eggs instead of deviled eggs
- Grilled Sirloin Steak
  with: house salad (no dressing, cheese, or croutons) or steamed vegetables
- 10 oz. Rib Eye Steak
  without: biscuits and muffins. side: house salad (no dressing, cheese, or croutons), steamed vegetables, or a plain baked potato (no cheese, sour cream, butter, bacon, etc.) optional: pepper, chives

Culver's

Drink: Water

Entrées

- Grilled Chicken Sandwich
  without: white bread (whole wheat/grain or lettuce bun instead)
- Garden Fresco with Grilled Chicken Salad
  without: dressing, cheese, and croutons
- Chicken Cashew With Grilled Chicken
  without: dressing, cheese, and croutons
- Vegetable Beef Soup
- Chicken Noodle Soup
  without noodles

Dairy Queen

Drink: Water

Sandwiches

- Grilled Chicken Sandwich
  without: white bread bun (whole wheat/grain or lettuce bun instead) and mayo

Salads

- Chicken BLT (Grilled Chicken)
- *without: dressing, bacon, and cheese*
- Side Salad
  without dressing

Sides

- Banana

Dave and Buster's

Drink: Water

Starter Salads & Soups

- Fresh Garden Salad
  without: cheese, tortilla strips, and dressing
- Southwestern Tortilla Soup
  without: cheese and tortilla strips

Salads

instead of dressing, ask for: lemon, pepper, vinegar, guacamole/avocados, or fresh salsa

- Grilled Chicken & Baby Kale
  without: dressing, cheese, and Parmesan crisp
- Grilled Steak Salad
  without: dressing, cheese, candied pecans, and frazzled onions

Handhelds

- California Smoked Turkey Melt
  without: white bread (instead, whole wheat/grain bread or a lettuce bun), caramelized onions, cheese, and aïoli

Remember:
Small changes make a huge difference.
Know that the small changes you make add up to make an amazing body through a realistic and physically painless process. Our small choices add up for the better!

Del Taco

Drink: Water

Handcrafted Salads

- Mexican Chopped Chicken Salad
  without: cheese, tortilla strips, and dressing

Street Tacos

with soft corn tortillas

- Carne Asada
  without roasted chile salsa
- Chicken
  without roasted chile salsa

Fresca Bowls

- Pollo Asado With Avocado
  without white rice (ask for lettuce instead)
- Avocado Veggie
  without white rice (ask for lettuce instead)

Remember:
Restaurant Survival Guide is intended to help readers lose body fat, and the Ocinator Fitness Program is intended to help users sculpt abs and other muscles.

Denny's

Drink: Water

Fit Fare

- Fit Slam
  without: turkey bacon and English muffin (unless the English muffin is whole wheat/grain). instead, ask for whole wheat/grain toast or more fruit
- Loaded Veggie Omelette
  without: cheese and English muffin (unless the English muffin is whole wheat/grain). instead, ask for whole wheat/grain toast or more fruit
- Tilapia Ranchero
  without butter on the corn
- Veggie Skillet
  ask for potatoes to be cooked with little to no oil
- Sirloin Steak
  without mashed potatoes. instead, ask for whole wheat toast or more vegetables

Soups

- Vegetable Beef Soup

Sandwiches & Salads

instead of dressing, ask for: lemon, pepper, vinegar, guacamole/avocados, or fresh salsa

- House Salad
  without: cheese, croutons, and dressing
- Tuscan Grilled Chicken Sandwich
- *without: white bread (whole wheat bun instead), bacon, cheese, and mayo*
- Avocado Chicken Caesar Salad
  without: bacon, cheese, and dressing

Denny's (2)

Drink: Water

<u>55+</u>

- 55+ Club Sandwich
  without: cheese, bacon, mayo, and fries
  ask for fruit or steamed vegetables instead of fries
- 55+ Grilled Tilapia
  with sides: steamed vegetables, whole wheat/grain toast, or fruit
- 55+ Grilled Chicken
  with sides: steamed vegetables, whole wheat/grain toast, or fruit

<u>Classics & Steaks</u>

- Mediterranean Grilled Chicken
  with sides: steamed vegetables, whole wheat/grain toast, or fruit
- Wild Alaska Salmon
  with sides of steamed vegetables, whole wheat/grain toast, or fruit
- T-Bone Steak
  with sides: steamed vegetables, whole wheat/grain toast, or fruit

Dickey's Barbecue Pit

Drink: Water

<u>Meat Plates</u>

- Sliced Beef Brisket, Chopped Beef Brisket, Chicken Breast, or Turkey
  sides: salad without dressing, cheese, and croutons
  without: white bread roll and sauce. get more salad instead

Domino's

Drink: Water

<u>Salads</u>

instead of dressing, ask for: lemon, pepper, vinegar, guacamole/avocados, or fresh salsa

- Classic Garden
  without: cheese and dressing
- Chicken Apple Pecan
  without: cheese and dressing

Einstein Bros Bagels

Drink: Water

<u>Classic</u>

- Ancient Grain (Plain)
  without: cream cheese, butter, jam, etc.

<u>Bread Specialty</u>

- Multigrain Roll (Plain)
  without cream cheese, butter, jam, etc.

Remember:

Stay away from refined grains.

The prominent advice in medicine today indicates how to lose weight healthily: stay away from products with *refined grain* and products with added sugar. Also, eat lots of vegetables. The key: *refined grain* carbs are bad. On the other hand, *whole grain* carbs are good.

El Pollo Loco

Drink: Water

Tacos

- Chicken Taco Al Carbon
- Chicken Avocado Taco
  without: cheese and dressing

Salads

- Double Chicken Avocado Salad
  without: sour cream and dressing
- Classic Salad
  without: tortilla strips and dressing
- Mexican Cobb Salad
  without: bacon, cheese, tortilla strips, and dressing

Bowls

- Pollo Bowl
  without: sour cream and dressing
- Grande Avocado
  without: tortilla strips and dressing
- Double Chicken Bowl
  without: bacon, cheese, tortilla strips, and dressing
- Chicken Black Bean Bowl
  without: bacon, cheese, tortilla strips, and dressing

Family Meals

- 8, 10, 12, or 16 Piece Meal
  sides: brown rice, black beans, broccoli, loco side salad (without tortilla strips, cheese, and dressing)

More Chicken

- Skinless Chicken Breast

Famous Dave's

Drink: Water

Salads 'N Soups

instead of dressing, ask for: lemon, pepper, vinegar, guacamole/avocados, or fresh salsa

- Chicken Chopped Salad
  without: cheese, tortilla strips, dressing, and corn bread muffin
  ask for whole wheat/grain bread or fruit as a substitute
- Fresh Garden Side Salad
  without: cheese, bacon, croutons, and dressing
  ask for whole wheat/grain bread or fruit as a substitute
- Mexican Cobb Salad
  without: bacon, cheese, tortilla strips, and dressing

Pitmaster Favorites

without corn bread muffin. for your two sides, see below

- Texas Beef Brisket
- Cedar Plank Salmon
  not glazed and caramelized. just grilled
- Country-Roasted Chicken

Side Dishes

- Fresh Steamed Broccoli
  sides: brown rice, black beans, broccoli, loco side salad (without tortilla strips, cheese, and dressing)
- Grilled Pineapple Steaks
  without: cayenne and sugar

Lunch

- Baked Potato
  without: cheese, bacon, sour cream, and butter.
  with (optional): pepper, green onions

Firehouse Subs

Drink: Water

Hot or Cold Specialty Subs

- Hook & Ladder
  without: white bread (whole wheat/grain bread instead), cheese, mayo, and mustard
- Firehouse Meatball
  without: white bread (whole wheat/grain bread instead) and cheese

Salads

instead of dressing, ask for: lemon, pepper, vinegar, guacamole/avocados, or fresh salsa

- Italian With Grilled Chicken Salad
  without: salami, cheese, and dressing
- Firehouse Salad
  without: cheese and dressing
- Hook & Ladder Salad
  without: cheese and dressing

Hot or Cold Subs

without cheese, mayo, mustard, and white bread (whole wheat/grain bread instead)

- Smoked Turkey Breast
- Grilled Chicken Breast
- Virginia Honey Ham

First Watch

Drink: Water

The Healthier Side

- Avocado Toast
- Healthy Turkey
  without feta
- Power Wrap
- Steel-Cut Oatmeal
  without: brown sugar and muffin
- Sunrise Granola Bowl
  without powdered sugar
- Tri-Athlete
  without: cheese and preserves

Omelets & Frittatas

- Inspired Italian Omelet
  without: sausage and cheese
- Morning Market Vegetable Omelet
  without: cheese and preserves

From The Griddle

- Multigrain Pancakes (Blueberry, Plain, or Banana Granola Crunch)
  without: butter, syrup, jam, and preserves

Power Bowls

- Pesto Chicken Quinoa Bowl
  without: pesto and feta
- Power Breakfast Bowl
  without: sausage, Parmesan, and olive oil. basted eggs with minimal oil, without butter

First Watch (2)

Drink: Water

<u>Salads</u>

instead of dressing, ask for: lemon, pepper, vinegar, guacamole/avocados, or fresh salsa

- Chicken Avocado Chop Salad
  without: cheese, tortilla chips, and dressing
- Cobb Salad
  without: bacon, cheese, and dressing
- Superfood Kale Salad
  without: Parmesan cheese and vinaigrette/dressing
- Sweet Honey Pecan Salad
  without: bacon, cheese, and honey dressing

<u>Sandwiches</u>

without white bread (whole wheat/grain bread instead)

- Market Veggie
  without: basil pesto, mayo, and cheese
- Monterey Club
  without: bacon, cheese, and mayo
- Baja Turkey Burger
  without: mayo and cheese
- Veggie Burger
  without: dijonnaise and cheese

<u>Juice</u>

- Kale Tonic Fresh Juice

<u>Sides</u>

- Whole Grain Artisan Toast
  without preserves
- Fresh Fruit
- Hearty Vegetable Soup
- Tomato Basil Soup

Five Guys Burgers and Fries

Drink: Water

<u>Burgers</u>

- Hamburger
  without: white bread (lettuce bun instead), mayo, mustard, ketchup, relish, bbq sauce, hot sauce, and a1 sauce

<u>Sandwiches</u>

- Veggie Sandwich
  without: white bread (lettuce bun instead), mayo, mustard, ketchup, relish, bbq sauce, hot sauce, and a1 sauce

<u>General Cuisine Guidelines</u>

American

Stay away from: fried food, cheese, sauce, dressing/ vinaigrette, and white bread/buns (including free appetizers).

Choose grilled and whole wheat options.

Fleming's Prime Steakhouse & Wine Bar

Drink: Water

Chef Curtis' Table

- Porterhouse Steak
  without bourbon bacon jam

Salads

instead of dressing, ask for: lemon, pepper, vinegar, guacamole/avocados, or fresh salsa

- Seasonal Salad
  without vinaigrette/dressing
- Wedge Salad
  without: bacon, cheese, and dressing

Sides

- Baked Potato (Plain)
  without: cheese, sour cream, butter, bacon, etc.
- Grilled High Country Asparagus

Signature Steaks

without butter

- Filet Mignon
- Prime New York Steak

Beyond Steak

- Double Breast of Chicken
- Barbecue Scottish Salmon Fillet
  without barbecue glaze

Freddy's Frozen Custard and Steakburgers

Drink: Water

Burgers

- Steakburger
  without: white bread (lettuce bun instead), cheese, mustard, ketchup, fries, chips and sauce

Sandwiches

- Grilled Chicken Breast Sandwich
  without: white bread, cheese, mustard, ketchup, fries, chips, and sauce

Be comfortable asking for:

- Whole grains, brown rice - instead of white/refined carbs*
- Food that is steamed, baked/grilled with no/minimal oil
- Lemon slices, vinegar, mustard, guacamole/avocados, or fresh salsa, pepper and other herbs - instead of dressings, condiments and sauces that contain extra oils/fats

*Including free appetizers

Hardee's

Drink: Water

Sandwiches

- Low Carb Charbroiled Chicken Club
  without: honey wheat bun (ask for a lettuce bun instead), bacon, cheese, and mayo

Salads

instead of dressing, ask for: lemon, pepper, vinegar, guacamole/avocados, or fresh salsa

- Charbroiled Chicken Salad
  without: cheese, croutons, and dressing
- Side Salad
  without: cheese, croutons, and dressing

Hungry Howie's

Drink: Water

Salads

instead of dressing, ask for: lemon, pepper, vinegar, guacamole/avocados, or fresh salsa

- Antipasto
  without: salami, cheese, and dressing
- Chef
  without: cheese and dressing
- Greek
  without: cheese and dressing
- Garden
  without: croutons and dressing
- Chicken Asiago
  without: cheese and dressing
- Chicken Caesar
  without: cheese and dressing

IHOP

Drink: Water or Low-Fat Milk

Omelettes

without butter

- Big Steak Omelette
  without: cheese and hash browns. with side of fruit or whole wheat/grain toast
- Chicken Fajita Omelette
  without: cheese and sour cream. side of fruit or whole wheat/grain toast
- Spinach & Mushroom Omelette
  without: cheese and hollandaise. side of fruit or whole wheat/grain toast
- Egg White Vegetable Omelette
  without cheese. with side of fruit or whole wheat/grain toast

Pancakes

- Harvest Grain 'N Nut
  without: butter, syrup, jam, preserves, etc. with side of fruit

Sandwiches

- Roasted Turkey Sandwich
  without: bacon, cheese, and mayonnaise

Salads

instead of dressing, ask for: lemon, pepper, vinegar, guacamole/avocados, or fresh salsa

- Grilled Chicken & Veggie Salad
  without vinaigrette/dressing
- Chicken Cobb Salad (Grilled Chicken)
  without: cheese and dressing
- House Salad
  without dressing

IHOP (2)

Drink: Water or Low-Fat Milk

Entrées

- Tilapia
  without: alfredo sauce and mashed potatoes. instead, ask for whole wheat/grain toast or fruit

In-N-Out

Drink: Water

Burgers

- Protein-Style Hamburger
  without: white bread bun (lettuce bun instead), cheese, and sauce without fries
- Protein-Style Double Meat
  without: white bread bun (lettuce bun instead), cheese, and sauce without fries

Remember:

Stay away from refined grains.

Refined grain carbs are unhealthy because they have been stripped of the nutrients that whole grains have. But because *whole grain* carbs have those nutrients, they are good for you.

Jamba Juice

Drink: Water

Fruit & Veggie Smoothies

- Apple 'n Greens Smoothie
- Greens 'n Ginger Smoothie
- Berry UpBEET Smoothie
- Apple 'n Greens Smoothie
- Orange Carrot Karma Smoothie

All Fruit Smoothies

- Mega Mango Smoothie
- Peach Perfection Smoothie
- Pomegranate Paradise Smoothie
- Strawberry Whirl Smoothie
- Orange Carrot Karma Smoothie

Bowls

- Peachy Green Goodness Bowl
- Fruit and Greek Yogurt Bowl

Tasty Bites

- Oatmeal

Protein Smoothies

- Fruit and Greek Yogurt Bowl

Boosts

- Greek Yogurt Boost
- Kale Boost
- Chia Seed Boost
- Chia Topper
- Pumpkin Seed Boost

Jason's Deli

Drink: Water

Specialty Sandwiches

instead of dressing, ask for: lemon, pepper, vinegar, guacamole/avocados, or fresh salsa

- Santa Fe Chicken Sandwich
  without: white bread (multigrain bread instead), bacon, cheese, and dressing
- MeataBalla
  without: French bread (whole wheat/grain bread instead) and cheese
- Amy's Turkey-O
  without: white bread (whole wheat/grain bread instead), cheese, and mustard
- JB's Southwest Turkey
  without: white bread (whole wheat/grain bread instead), cheese, and aïoli

Wraps

- Turkey Wrap
  without ranch. with side of fruit or steamed veggies
- Mediterranean Wrap
  without hummus. with side of fruit or steamed veggies
- Ranchero Wrap
  without cheddar jalapeños. with side of fruit or steamed veggies

Famous Favorites

- Wild Salmon-wich
  without: white bread (whole wheat/grain bread instead) and aïoli
  with side of fruit or steamed veggies

Soups

- Organic Vegetable
- Tomato Basil

Jason's Deli (2)

Drink: Water

Build Your Own Sandwich

instead of dressing, ask for: lemon, pepper, vinegar, guacamole/avocados, or fresh salsa

- Meats
  Ham, Roasted Turkey Breast, Smoked Turkey Breast, Pineapple
- Breads
  Multigrain Wheat, Rye, Gluten-Free Bread, Organic Wheat Wrap, Organic Ancient Grain Bun
  without: white bread, white flour tortilla
- Add-Ons
  Guacamole, Avocado Slices
- Spreads and Cheeses
  without spreads and cheese (vinegar and/or pepper instead)

Salads

instead of dressing, ask for: lemon, pepper, vinegar, guacamole/avocados, or fresh salsa

- Chicken Club Salad
  without: bacon, cheese, dressing
- Nutty Mixed-Up Salad
  without: cheese and dressing
- Mesa Chicken Salad
  without: cheese and dressing
- Salmon Pacifica Salad
  without vinaigrette/dressing
- The Big Chef
  without cheese

Potatoes

- Pollo Mexicano Potato
  without: cheese, sour cream, and butter

Jason's Deli (3)

Drink: Water

<u>Meatless Eats</u>

- Spinach Veggie Wrap
  without: white flour wrap (whole wheat/grain wrap instead) and cheese
  with side of fruit, steamed veggies, or baked chips
- Fresh Fruit
  without creamy dip
- Zucchini Grillini
  ask for bread to have very little olive oil
  without white bread (whole wheat/grain bread instead) and cheese
  with side of fruit, steamed veggies, or baked chips
- Black Bean Taco Salad
  without: blue corn chips (unless baked), cheese, and sour cream. ask for baked chips, steamed veggies, or fruit instead of blue corn chips

Jet's Pizza

Drink: Water

<u>Salads</u>

instead of dressing, ask for: lemon, pepper, vinegar, guacamole/avocados, or fresh salsa

- Antipasto Salad
  without: salami, cheese, and dressing
- Garden Salad
  without: cheese and dressing
- Greek Salad
  without: cheese and dressing
- Chicken Caesar Salad
  without: Parmesan, croutons, and dressing

Jersey Mike's Subs

Drink: Water

<u>Cold Subs</u>

with whole wheat/grain bread (without white bread)
without: cheese, mayo, olive oil, and white bread
instead of dressing, ask for: lemon, pepper, vinegar, guacamole/avocados, or fresh salsa

- #3 The American Classic (Ham)
- #14 The Veggie
- #7 Turkey Breast
- #6 Famous Roast Beef
- #8 Cold Sub (Turkey & Ham)

Remember:
Stay away from products with added sugar and artificial sweeteners.
Stay away from: soda, most desserts, dressings, syrups, jams, jellies, etc. Instead, try eating naturally sweet food like fruit.

Jimmy John's Gourmet Sandwiches

Drink: Water

Classics

with whole wheat/grain bread (without white bread)
without: white bread, dijon, cheese, mayo, and olive oil
instead of dressing, ask for: lemon, pepper, vinegar, guacamole/avocados, or fresh salsa

- #2 Original Roast Beef
- #4 Turkey Breast
- #1 Ham
- #6 Veggie

Favorites

with whole wheat/grain bread (without white bread)
without: dijon, cheese, mayo, and white bread
instead of dressing, ask for: lemon, pepper, vinegar, guacamole/avocados, or fresh salsa

- #8 Roast Beef & Ham
- #10 Double Roast Beef
- #14 Roast Beef & Turkey Breast
- #7 Double Ham
- #11 Turkey & Ham
- #13 Veggie Club

KFC

Drink: Water

Grilled Chicken

- 8, 12, and 16 pc. Bucket Meal
  without biscuits. ask to substitute side below instead of biscuits

Sides

- Green Beans
- Corn (if available without butter)

Remember:

Stay away from refined grains.

Studies have shown that not eating whole grain carbs could lead to: poorer memory-based task performance, bad breath, and increased anger, depression, anxiety, irritability, and hostility.

Logan's Roadhouse

- Drink: Water

Salads & Soups

instead of dressing, ask for: lemon, pepper, vinegar, guacamole/avocados, or fresh salsa

- Mesquite Grilled Chicken Salad
  without: cheese, croutons, and dressing
- Roadhouse Steak Cobb Salad
  without: bacon, cheese, croutons, and dressing
- Fresh Garden Salad
  without: cheese, croutons, and dressing

Sides

- Baked Potato (Plain)
  without: cheese, sour cream, butter, bacon, etc.
- Steamed Broccoli
- Fresh Garden Salad
  without: cheese, croutons, and dressing
- Roasted Corn Salad (Seasonal Special)
  without: vinaigrette and cheese
- Corn
  without butter

Burgers & Sandwiches

without fries or chips. see sides above for substitutes

- Logan's Club
  without: white bread (whole wheat/grain bread or a lettuce bun instead), bacon, cheese, and mayo
- Grilled Chicken Sandwich
  without: white bread (whole wheat/grain bread or a lettuce bun instead), bacon, cheese, and mayo

Logan's Roadhouse (2)

Drink: Water

Chicken & Seafood

see sides section above

- Logan's Wood-Grilled Chicken
  without: Parmesan peppercorn dressing and white rice. ask for more salad without dressing instead
- Mesquite Wood-Grilled Salmon
  without: white rice and sauce. ask for more salad without dressing instead
- Lemon Herb Chicken
  without: butter and white rice. ask for more salad without dressing instead

Steak

- Top Sirloin
  without mayo
- Filet Mignon
  without: white bread, cheese, and olive oil
- New York Strip
  without: white bread, cheese, and olive oil

Long John Silver's

Drink: Water

Baked Meals

- Baked Cod Meal
  without: white rice and hushpuppies. ask for steamed vegetables or a salad without dressing, croutons, or cheese instead

Longhorn Steakhouse

Drink: Water

Legendary Steaks

get double salad (without dressing, cheese, croutons) instead of a side. also, don't eat the steak fat

- Renegade Sirloin
  without butter
- Outlaw Ribeye
  without butter
- New York Strip
  without butter
- Flat Iron Steak
  without butter
- Fire-Grilled T-Bone
  without butter
- The Longhorn
  without butter

Salad

instead of dressing, ask for: lemon, pepper, vinegar, guacamole/avocados, or fresh salsa

- Grilled Chicken & Strawberry Salad
  without: candied pecans, feta, and raspberry vinaigrette
- 7-Pepper Sirloin Salad
  without: cheese, croutons, and dressing

Sides

- Mixed Green Salad
  without: dressing, croutons, and cheese
- 7-Pepper Sirloin Salad
  without: cheese, croutons, and dressing

Maggiano's Little Italy

Drink: Water

Salad

instead of dressing, ask for: lemon, pepper, vinegar, guacamole/avocados, or fresh salsa

- Italian Tossed Salad
  without: pepperoncini, croutons, and vinaigrette/dressing
- Grilled Salmon Salad
  without: croutons, cheese, and vinaigrette/dressing
- Grilled Chicken Salad
  without: mozzarella, croutons, and vinaigrette/dressing

Sides

- Fresh Grilled Asparagus
  without: cheese, croutons, and vinaigrette/dressing

On The House Classic Pastas

get whole wheat penne. or gluten-free if you have gluten sensitivities

- Whole Wheat Penne with Marinara
- Whole Wheat Penne with Meatball
- Whole Wheat Penne with Meat Sauce

Seafood

- Grilled Salmon Lemon & Herb
  without white wine butter sauce

Chicken

- Grilled Chicken (a la carte)

Maggiano's Little Italy (2)

Drink: Water

<u>Steak & Veal</u>

- Filet Mignon
  without asparagus risotto. ask for grilled or steamed asparagus instead
- Center-Cut Filet Mignon
  without: garlic butter and crispy vesuvio potatoes. ask for steamed or grilled potatoes instead

Marco's Pizza

Drink: Water

<u>Salads</u>

instead of dressing, ask for: lemon, pepper, vinegar, guacamole/avocados, or fresh salsa

- Antipasto
  without: salami, cheese, and dressing
- Chicken Caesar
  without: Parmesan cheese, croutons, and dressing
- Greek
  without: feta cheese and dressing
- Garden
  without: cheddar cheese, croutons, and dressing

McAlister's Deli

Drink: Water

Sandwiches

with whole wheat/grain bread and wraps
without white bread or white flour wraps
instead of dressing, ask for: lemon, pepper, vinegar, guacamole/avocados, or fresh salsa

- The McAlister's Club
  without: white bread, bacon, cheddar, Swiss, mayo, and mustard
- King Club
  without: white bread, bacon, cheddar, Swiss, mayo, and mustard
- McAlister's Club Wrap
  without: white flour wrap, bacon, cheddar, Swiss, mayo, and mustard
- Black Angus Club
  without: white bread, bacon, cheddar, Swiss, mayo, and horseradish sauce
- Grilled Chicken Club
  without: white bread, bacon, cheddar, Swiss, mayo, and honey mustard sauce
- Turkey Cobb
  without: white bread, bacon, cheese, mayo, and ranch
- Garden Fresh Turkey
  without: white bread, cheese, and vinaigrette
- The Veggie
  without: white bread and mayo

Soups

- Fire Roasted Vegetable
- Chicken Tortilla
  without: cheese and tortilla strips
- Tomato Bisque

McAlister's Deli (2)

Drink: Water

<u>Salads</u>

instead of dressing, ask for: lemon, pepper, vinegar, guacamole/avocados, or fresh salsa

- Savannah Chopped Salad
  without: honey roasted almonds, gorgonzola, and dressing
- Southwest Cobb
  without: cheese, tortilla chips, and dressing
- Italian Chopped Salad
  without: salami, cheese, and dressing
- Grilled Chicken Salad
  without: cheese, croutons, and dressing
- Grilled Chicken Salad
  without: cheese, croutons, and dressing
- Chef Salad
  without: bacon, cheese, croutons, and dressing
- Garden Salad
  without: cheese, croutons, and dressing

Remember:
Eating whole grain carbs could lead to positive effects by allowing the soluble fiber, found in whole grain carbs, to:

- Decrease LDL (bad) cholesterol
- Increase good HDL cholesterol
- Increase dietary fiber
- Help promote fat loss
- Prevent fat gain
- Lower the risk of diabetes

McDonald's

Drink: Water

Sandwiches

- Artisan Grilled Chicken Sandwich
  without: white bread (lettuce bun instead) and sauce

Salads

instead of dressing, ask for: lemon, pepper, vinegar, guacamole/avocados, or fresh salsa

- Bacon and Ranch Grilled Chicken Salad
  without: bacon, ranch, and cheese
- Southwest Grilled Chicken Salad
  without: cheese, tortilla strips, dressing, and cilantro lime glaze
- Side Salad
  without dressing

Sides

- Kids' Apple Slices

Remember:
Stay away from products with added sugar and artificial sweeteners.
The more you stay away from products with added sugar, the sweeter naturally sweet food, like fruit, will taste!

Mellow Mushroom

Drink: Water

Salads

instead of dressing, ask for: lemon, pepper, vinegar, guacamole/avocados, or fresh salsa

- Greek Salad
  without feta cheese
- House Salad
  without: Parmesan cheese and vinaigrette/dressing
- Chef Salad
  without: mozzarella, provolone, and dressing

Munchies

- Meatball Trio
  without: mozzarella, Parmesan, and breadcrumbs

Sandwiches & Hoagies

- Chicken Caesar Wrap
  without: white flour wrap (multigrain wrap instead) and sauce
- Country Club
  without: white bread (multigrain bread instead) and sauce
- California Club
  without: white bread (multigrain bread instead) and sauce
- Avocado Hoagie
  without: white bread (multigrain roll instead), provolone, and mayo
- Meatball Hoagie
  without: white bread (multigrain roll instead) and mozzarella

Miller's Ale House

Drink: Water

On The Greens

instead of dressing, ask for: lemon, pepper, vinegar, guacamole/avocados, or fresh salsa

- Asian Grilled Chicken Salad
  without: crispy rice noodles and sesame-ginger vinaigrette
- Blackened Chicken Breast Salad
  without: cheese, crispy tortilla strips, garlic-lime crema, and vinaigrette/dressing
- House Salad
  without: cheese, croutons, and vinaigrette/dressing
- Southwest Seared Flat Iron Steak Salad
  without: cheese, crispy onion tanglers, Dijon-horseradish drizzle, and vinaigrette/dressing

Two Hand Grip

- Grilled Chicken Breast Sandwich
  without brioche bun (lettuce bun instead). with guacamole and fresh pico de gallo
- Mahi-Mahi Sandwich
  without: brioche bun (lettuce bun instead) and tartar sauce

From The Grill

with steamed vegetables

- Center Cut Sirloin
- Flat Iron Steak
- Filet Mignon
- Ribeye

Miller's Ale House (2)

Drink: Water

From The Sea

with steamed vegetables

- Atlantic Salmon
  without: coleslaw and tartar sauce
- Mahi-Mahi
  without: coleslaw and tartar sauce
- North Atlantic Lobster Tail
  without butter

Fajitas

with grilled (not sautéed) vegetables
without cheese, sour cream, flour tortillas

- Grilled Marinated Chicken Breast
- Grilled Flat Iron Steak
- Steak and Chicken Combo

Sides

- Baked Potato
  without: butter, sour cream, etc.
- Seasonal Vegetable
  steamed or grilled
- Beans

Moe's Southwest Grill

Drink: Water

Burritos

- Homewrecker Mexican Burrito With Guac (Steak, Chicken, Fish, or Tofu)
  without: white flour tortilla (whole wheat/grain tortilla instead), white rice, cheese, sour cream, ranch, vinaigrette, bacon, and queso
- Joey Southwest Burrito (Steak, Chicken, Fish, or Tofu)
  without: white flour tortilla (whole wheat/grain tortilla instead), white rice, cheese, sour cream, ranch, vinaigrette, bacon, and queso

Bowls

- Bowl'd Southwest Flavors Earmuffs (Steak, Chicken, Fish, or Tofu)
  without: white rice, cheese, sour cream, ranch, vinaigrette, bacon, and queso.

Tacos

- Steak or Chicken
  without: avocado lime crema, queso fresco, slaw, sour cream, ranch, vinaigrette, bacon, and queso. with soft corn tortilla

Salads

instead of dressing, ask for: lemon, pepper, vinegar, guacamole/avocados, or fresh salsa

- Chicken, Steak, Fish, or Tofu
  without: avocado lime crema, queso fresco, slaw, sour cream, ranch, vinaigrette, bacon, and queso. don't eat the hard shell (fried) bowl

Sides

- Pico de Gallo
- Guacamole

Moe's Southwest Grill (2)

Drink: Water

Stacks

- Steak, Chicken, Fish, or Tofu
  without: white flour tortilla (whole grain tortilla instead), fried hard corn tortillas (soft corn tortillas instead) white rice, cheese, sour cream, ranch, vinaigrette, bacon, and queso

Remember:
Stay away from products with added sugar and artificial sweeteners.
Look out for hidden sugars and additives. For example, dressing contains too much added sugar, as well as saturated fat and sodium that can lead to increased body fat and feelings of hunger.

Ninety Nine Restaurant & Pub

Drink: Water

Burgers

with steamed vegetables or side salad without dressing

- West Coast Turkey Burger
  without: white bread (whole wheat/grain bun/bread or lettuce bun instead) and cheese
- Vegetarian Black Bean Burger
  without: white bread (whole wheat/grain bun/bread or lettuce bun instead) and dressing (on salad)
- Burger
  without: white bread (whole wheat/grain bun/bread or lettuce bun instead) and cheese

Sandwiches

- Triple-Decker Turkey Club
  without: bacon and cheese

9.99

see below for sides

- Grilled Chicken
  without balsamic glaze
- Grilled Ribeye Steak
  without bacon marmalade
- Chopped Grilled Angus
  without: mashed potatoes, red wine sauce, sautéed mushrooms, and crispy onions. ask for grilled or steamed vegetables instead

Ninety Nine Restaurant & Pub (2)

Drink: Water

Salads

instead of dressing, ask for: lemon, pepper, vinegar, guacamole/avocados, or fresh salsa

- Sundried Tomato Chicken Kabob Salad
  without: feta cheese, croutons, and dressing
- Sirloin Tip Heart of Caesar Salad
  without: Caesar dressing, bacon, croutons, and Parmesan cheese

Chicken, Turkey & More

with steamed vegetables or side salad without dressing

- Grilled Turkey Tip Skewers
  without: white bread (whole wheat/grain bun/bread or lettuce instead), sauce, and vinaigrette/dressing

Seafood

see sides section for side choices

- Fresh Salmon
  without feta cheese

Gluten Sensitive

see above for duplicates. sides: in-season vegetable (grilled or steamed) or baked potato (plain)

- Fresh Seasoned Salmon
- Royal Sirloin
  without cheese and dressing on salad
- Broiled Sirloin Tips
  without cheese and dressing on salad

Ninety Nine Restaurant & Pub (3)

- Drink: Water

Gluten Sensitive Side Salads

- Heart of Caesar Side Salad
  without: bacon, croutons, and dressing
- Garden Side Salad
  without: Parmesan, croutons, and dressing

Steaks and Ribs

- Royal Sirloin
  without cheese and dressing on salad
- Broiled Sirloin Tips
  without cheese and dressing on salad
- Top Sirloin Steak
  without cheese and dressing on salad

Remember:
Stay away from products with added sugar and artificial sweeteners.
Research changes regarding the side effects of artificial sweeteners, so it is best to avoid them.

Noodles World Kitchen

Drink: Water

Veggie Noodles

- Zucchini with Grilled Chicken
  without: sauce, cream, and cheese
- Zucchini Romesco
  without: red pepper sauce, cream, and feta

Salads

instead of dressing, ask for: lemon, pepper, vinegar, guacamole/avocados, or fresh salsa

- The Med Salad With Chicken
  without: spicy yogurt dressing, cavatappi pasta (if possible, ask for zucchini pasta instead), and feta
- Chicken Veracruz Salad
  without: chili-lime chicken (grilled chicken instead), bacon, dressing, and crispy jalapeños
- Grilled Chicken Caesar
  without: dressing, croutons, and Parmesan

Soups

- Tomato Basil Bisque
- Chicken Noodle Soup
  without noodles (or with plain zucchini noodles, if possible)

Sides

- Tomato Basil Bisque
- Chicken Noodle Soup
  without noodles
- Tossed Green Side Salad
  without: vinaigrette/dressing
- Caesar Side Salad
  without: dressing, croutons, and Parmesan

O'Charley's

Drink: Water

Soups, Salads, and Sides

instead of dressing, ask for: lemon, pepper, vinegar, guacamole/avocados, or fresh salsa

- Southern Pecan Chicken Tender Salad
  without: dried cranberries, cheese, candied pecans, and dressing/vinaigrette
- Sonoma Chicken Salad
  without: dressing and bbq sauce
- California Chicken Salad
  without: cheese, candied pecans, dried cranberries, and dressing/vinaigrette
- The Classic Cobb
  without: cheese, bacon, croutons, and dressing/vinaigrette
- Steakhouse Wedge Salad
  without: cheese and dressing/vinaigrette
- Chicken Tortilla Soup
  without: cheese and tortilla strips
- Chicken Harvest Soup
  without: cheese
- Fresh Broccoli
- Baked Potato (Plain)
  without: butter, sour cream, cheese, bacon, etc.
- Fresh Grilled Asparagus

Over The Top And Under $10

- Chopped Steak
  without gravy, fried onions, and bacon smashed potatoes. ask for sides from above instead
- Santa Fe Tilapia
  without white rice. ask for a side from above instead

O'Charley's (2)

Drink: Water

Sunday Brunch

without white bread toast (whole wheat/grain bread instead)

- Veggie Omelet
  without: cheese, butter, oil, and Parmesan potatoes (ask for more fruit or toast instead)
- Country Scramble
  without: cheese, butter, oil, sausage, bacon, and Parmesan potatoes (ask for more fruit or toast instead)
- Ultimate Omelet
  without: cheese, butter, oil, and Parmesan potatoes (ask for a side from above instead)

Fresh Burgers & Sandwiches

instead of fries: fresh broccoli, baked potato, fresh grilled asparagus, or fruit

- The Club Sandwich
  without: white bread (whole wheat/grain bread instead), bacon, cheese, mayo, and honey mustard

Steaks, Ribs, & Prime Rib

sides: fresh broccoli, baked potato, fresh grilled asparagus, or fruit

- Grilled Top Sirloin
- Filet Mignon
  without garlic butter

Seafood Favorites

sides: fresh broccoli, baked potato, fresh grilled asparagus, or fruit

- Fresh Cedar-Planked Salmon
- Fresh Grilled Atlantic Salmon

Classic Combos

sides: fresh broccoli, baked potato, fresh grilled asparagus, or fruit

- Steak & Grilled Atlantic Salmon

Olive Garden

Drink: Water

Note: don't eat breadsticks (made with white bread)

Soups & Salads

instead of dressing, ask for: lemon, pepper, vinegar, guacamole/avocados, or fresh salsa

- ToGo Our Famous House Salad
  without: cheese, dressing, and croutons
- Minestrone
- Unlimited Our Famous House Salad
  without: cheese, dressing, and croutons

Cucina Mia! – Create Your Own Pasta Bowl

- Whole Grain Linguine
  with: traditional marinara or traditional meat sauce; meatballs, grilled chicken, or garden veggies
- Gluten-Free Rotini
  with: traditional marinara or traditional meat sauce; meatballs, grilled chicken, or garden veggies

Tastes Of The Mediterranean

- Salmon Piccata
  without: garlic butter sauce and Parmesan-crusted zucchini (ask for grilled vegetables instead)
- Herb-Grilled Salmon
  without: garlic butter sauce and Parmesan-crusted zucchini (ask for grilled vegetables instead)

Olive Garden (2)

- Drink: Water

Chicken

- Chicken Giardino
  with: whole wheat pasta instead of pappardelle pasta. or gluten-free pasta if you have gluten sensitivities
  without: bacon, cheese, mayo, honey mustard, and white bread (ask for grilled vegetables instead)
- Chicken Piccata
  without: garlic butter sauce and Parmesan-crusted zucchini (ask for grilled vegetables instead)

Beef

- 6 oz Sirloin
  without: garlic butter, Parmesan-crusted zucchini (ask for grilled vegetables instead), fettuccine alfredo (instead, whole wheat pasta, or gluten-free pasta if you have gluten sensitivities, and marinara or meat sauce)

Remember:
Stay away from products with added sugar and artificial sweeteners.
Small changes like eating fruit and getting rid of salad dressing add up and make a huge difference!

On The Border

Drink: Water

Starters

- Guacamole

Soup & Salads

instead of dressing, ask for: lemon, pepper, vinegar, guacamole/avocados, or fresh salsa

- Chicken Tortilla Soup
  without: cheese and tortilla strips
- Grande Taco Salad
  without: cheese, sour cream sauce, flour tortilla crisps, and dressing
- Fajita Salad
  ask for fajitas to be cooked with little to no oil
  without queso fresco and dressing
- Mango Chicken Salad
  without: queso fresco, vinaigrette, and dressing

Tacos

- Southwest Chicken Tacos
  without: flour tortillas (soft corn tortillas instead), cheese, creamy red chile sauce, and fried onion strings
- Street-Style Mini Tacos (Steak or Chicken)
  without: sautéed onion and cheese
- Grilled Fish Tacos Del Mar
  without: chimichurri, lime cabbage-carrot slaw, and mayo

Fajitas

with soft corn tortillas instead of flour tortillas, beans, pico de gallo, and guacamole. without rice (extra of one of the options above instead)

- Classic Fajitas (Chicken, Steak, or Portobello & Vegetables)
  ask for fajitas to be cooked with little to no oil

On The Border (2)

Drink: Water

Favorites

instead of rice, ask for grilled vegetables or beans without cheese

- Grilled Fiesta Chicken
  without: queso, sautéed vegetables, and rice
- Mexican Grilled Chicken
  without rice
- Carne Asada
  without rice

Border Bowls

- Border Bowls (Chicken or Steak without chimichurri)
  without: rice and queso

Sides

- Black Beans
  without cheese
- Refried Beans
  without cheese
- Corn Tortillas
- Guacamole
- Avocado Slices
- Taco (Chicken Tinga or Beef)
  with soft corn tortilla
  without: white flour tortilla and cheese

Party Platters

- Tacos (Chicken Tinga or Beef)
  with soft corn tortillas
  without cheese

On The Border (3)

Drink: Water

Family Meals

- Fajita Family Meal (Chicken or Steak)
  without: flour tortillas (get soft corn tortillas instead), sour cream, and cheese. ask for fajitas to be cooked with little to no oil
- Taco Family Meal (Chicken Tinga or Beef)
  with soft corn tortillas
  without cheese

Remember:

Balance your meats.

Though this book lists beef menu options, it is not a free pass to eat beef during every meal. Try eating mostly chicken and fish. Consuming too much red meat can be unhealthy.

Outback Steakhouse

Drink: Water

Starters

- Guacamole

Soups & Side Salads

instead of dressing, ask for: lemon, pepper, vinegar, guacamole/avocados, or fresh salsa

- Chicken Tortilla Soup
  without: cheese and tortilla strips
- House Salad
  without: dressing, cheese, and croutons

Lunch Sides

- Baked Potato (Plain)
  without: butter, cheese, sour cream, bacon, etc.
- Sweet Potato (Plain)
  without: honey butter and brown sugar
- Grilled Asparagus
  without olive oil

Signature Steaks

with plain baked potato, salad, and side from above

- Outback Center-Cut Sirloin
- Victoria's Filet Mignon
  without: queso, sautéed vegetables, and white rice (ask for grilled vegetables or beans without cheese instead)
- Ribeye

Outback Steakhouse (2)

Drink: Water

Chicken, Ribs, Chops & More

- Grilled Chicken On The Barbie
  without bbq sauce
- Perfectly Grilled Salmon
  without bbq sauce
- Simply Grilled Tilapia
  without bbq sauce

Steak And Lobster

- Victoria's Filet Mignon & Lobster
  without butter
- Bone-In Natural Cut Ribeye
  without: butter, cheese, sour cream, and bacon on potato

Walkabout Wednesday

without fries. instead: plain baked potato, salad, or side from above (they might charge extra)

- 6 Oz Center-Cut Sirloin
- Grilled Chicken On The Barbie

Steak Mates

- Steamed Lobster Tail
  without butter
- Perfectly Grilled Salmon
- *without bbq sauce*
- Simply Grilled Tilapia
  without bbq sauce

Panda Express

Drink: Water

<u>Sides</u>

- Mixed Vegetables
- Brown Steamed Rice

Panera Bread

Drink: Water

<u>Soups</u>

- Low-Fat Chicken Noodle Soup
- Black Bean Soup

<u>Salads</u>

instead of dressing, ask for: lemon, pepper, vinegar, guacamole/avocados, or fresh salsa

- Strawberry Poppyseed Salad With Chicken
  without: dressing and oil roasted pecans
- Asian Sesame Salad with Chicken
  without: Asian sesame vinaigrette and wonton strips
- Southwest Chile Lime Ranch Salad with Chicken
  without: masa chips, dressing, and feta
- Modern Greek Salad with Quinoa
  without: dressing and feta
- Green Goddess Cobb Salad with Chicken
  without: pickled onions, dressing, mayonnaise, and bacon
- Fuji Apple Salad with Chicken
  without: dressing, apple chips, oil roasted pecans, and Gorgonzola
- Greek Salad
  without: feta and dressing
- Caesar Salad with Chicken
  without: Parmesan, croutons, and dressing
- Seasonal Greens Salad
  without vinaigrette/dressing

Panera Bread (2)

Drink: Water

Sandwiches

- Turkey Sandwich (whole or half)
  without: mayo and mustard
- Ham Sandwich
  without: Swiss, mayo, and mustard
- Mediterranean Veggie Sandwich
  without: tomato basil bread (whole wheat/grain bread instead), feta, and hummus
- Roasted Turkey & Avocado BLT
  without white bread (whole wheat/grain bread instead), bacon, and mayo

Breakfast Sandwiches

- Avocado, Egg White & Spinach
  without: bagel (ask for whole wheat/grain bread instead) and cheddar
- Ham & Egg
  without cheese

Freshly Baked Breads

- Rye
- Whole Grain

Papa John's

Drink: Water

Papa's Salads

instead of dressing, ask for: lemon, pepper, vinegar, guacamole/avocados, or fresh salsa

- Papa's Garden Salad
  without: dressing, croutons, and cheese
- Chicken Caesar Salad
  without: cheese, croutons, and Caesar dressing

Pappadeaux Seafood Kitchen

Drink: Water

Soups & Salads

instead of dressing, ask for: lemon, pepper, vinegar, guacamole/avocados, or fresh salsa

- Pappas Greek Salad
  without: feta cheese and dressing
- Pappadeaux House Salad
  without: croutons, bacon, cheddar, and dressing
- Classic Caesar
  without: croutons, Parmesan cheese, and Caesar dressing
- Chopped Salad (with Grilled Salmon)
  without: bacon, cheese, vinaigrette, fried chicken, and fried crawfish
- Seafood Cobb Salad
  without: bacon, cheese, and vinaigrette/dressing

Chef Selections

- Rainbow Trout & Shrimp
  without: butter sauce and sautéed spinach (ask for grilled spinach or other vegetable instead)
- Halibut & Spanish Octopus
  without butter sauce
- Grilled Tilapia & Jumbo Shrimp
  without butter
- Grilled Redfish & Jumbo Shrimp
  without: butter and risotto
- Atlantic Salmon Yvette
  without: white wine sauce and white rice (ask for grilled vegetables or a salad without dressing, cheese, and croutons instead)

Pappadeaux Seafood Kitchen (2)

Drink: Water

<u>Steak, Lobster & Crab</u>

- Prime Beef Rib-Eye
  without: mashed potatoes (and ask for broccolini to be steamed or grilled, not sautéed)
- Filet Mignon
  without: butter and mashed potatoes (and ask for asparagus to be steamed or grilled, not sautéed)
- Filet Mignon & Grilled Rock Lobster
  without: butter and mashed potatoes
- Grilled Caribbean Lobster Tail
  without: butter and mashed potatoes (and ask for broccolini to be steamed or grilled, not sautéed)

Remember:
Eat lots of vegetables.
We all know the many benefits of eating most vegetables! Fiber and vitamins and minerals help us look and feel fresh.

Pei Wei Asian Diner

Drink: Water

<u>Small Plates, Shareables & Soups</u>

- Edamame
  without: feta cheese and dressing

<u>Chef Selections</u>

instead of dressing, ask for: lemon, pepper, vinegar, guacamole/avocados, or fresh salsa

- Kale Quinoa Chicken Salad
  without: tangy Asian slaw, vinaigrette, and dressing
- Ahi Avocado Salad
  without: Asian slaw, pickled ginger, crispy wontons, wasabi vinaigrette, and dressing
- Asian Chopped Chicken Salad
  without: crispy wontons, vinaigrette, and dressing
- Miso Side Salad
  without: miso ginger and side dressing

Perkins Restaurant & Bakery

Drink: Water

<u>Farm Fresh Omelets</u>

- Hearty Harvest
  without: turkey sausage and feta cheese
- Build-Your-Own
  without cheese
  with two of the following: ham, crimini mushrooms, tomatoes, spinach, fresh broccoli, fresh avocado, onions, green peppers. dry whole wheat toast or fruit on the side

<u>Perfect Platters</u>

- Potato Pancakes
  without: butter, applesauce, bacon strips
  ask for fresh fruit as a side

<u>Build-A-Breakfast</u>

- Eggs
  with grilled ham, fresh fruit, and whole wheat toast (without butter)

<u>Salads & Soups</u>

instead of dressing, ask for: lemon, pepper, vinegar, guacamole/avocados, or fresh salsa

- Southwest Avocado
  without: cheese, tortilla straws, and dressing
- The Chopped Cobb
  without: bacon, feta cheese, and dressing
- Tomato Basil Soup
  without croutons
- Chicken Tortilla Soup
  without: tortilla strips, cheese, and sour cream

Perkins Restaurant & Bakery (2)

Drink: Water

<u>Sides</u>

- Garden Salad
  without: cheese, croutons, and dressing
- Fresh Fruit
- Grilled Summer Vegetables
- Fresh Broccoli
- Baked Potato (Plain)
  without: butter, cheese, bacon, sour cream, etc.

<u>Comfort Classics</u>

- Grilled Chicken With Mushrooms and Asparagus
  without: white rice (brown rice okay), vinaigrette, sauce, and sautéed mushrooms (grilled mushrooms instead)
- Butterball Turkey (see above for sides)
  without: gravy, cranberry sauce, and dressing

<u>Burgers</u>

- Hamburger
  with only: beef patty, lettuce, tomato, egg (ask to be cooked with little to no oil)
  without white bread bun (whole wheat/grain bread or lettuce bun instead)

<u>Half Sandwiches</u>

- Turkey & Avocado
  without: bacon and aïoli
- Roast Beef
  without: French roll (whole wheat bread instead), cheese, and aïoli

P.F. Chang's

Drink: Water

Salads & Soups

instead of dressing, ask for: lemon, pepper, vinegar, guacamole/avocados, or fresh salsa

- Asian Caesar Salad (Chicken, Shrimp, or Salmon)
  without: Parmesan, wonton croutons, and dressing
- Mandarin Crunch Salad (Chicken, Shrimp, or Salmon)
  without: crispy rice sticks and vinaigrette/dressing
- Egg Drop Soup

Sushi

- Ahi Poke Bowl
  without: mandarin vinaigrette and wonton crisps
- Lobster Avocado Roll (if brown rice is available)
  without: white rice (brown rice instead) and curry aïoli

Main Entrees – Chicken, Beef, or Fish

- Chicken, Beef, or Fish With Steamed Broccoli
  ask for the chicken, beef, or fish to be grilled or cooked with little to no oil. without sauce
  with side: steamed brown rice

Main Entrees – Vegetarian

- Buddha's Feast
  without sauce. and ask for vegetables to be steamed or cooked with little to no oil
  side: steamed brown rice

Poke (General)

- Drink: Water

<u>Base</u>

- Brown Rice
- Spring Mix
- Kale

<u>Fish</u>

- Tuna
- Salmon
- Albacore
- Yellowtail
- Shrimp
- Octopus

<u>Sides</u>

- Crabmeat
- Avocado
- Edamame

<u>Toppings</u>

- Green Onion
- Cucumber
- Sprouts
- Cilantro
- Smelt Eggs
- Red Onion
- Tomato
- Serrano Pepper
- Pineapple

Pollo Tropical

Drink: Water

Sides

- Brown Rice
- Black Beans
- Caesar Salad (with Grilled Chicken Breast)
  without: Caesar dressing, croutons, Parmesan cheese, and Pollo Bites
- Red Beans
- Brown Rice & Black Beans

Salads & Soup

instead of dressing, ask for: lemon, pepper, vinegar, guacamole/avocados, or fresh salsa

- Mango Chicken Salad (grilled chicken breast)
  without: candied walnuts, Pollo Bites, and vinaigrette/dressing
- Caesar Salad (grilled chicken breast)
  without: caesar dressing, croutons, Parmesan cheese, and Pollo Bites
- Caribbean Chicken Soup

TropiChop Bowls

- Chicken or Vegetarian (no sauce)
  with only: steamed or grilled vegetables (no butter), brown rice, romaine lettuce (no dressing), or ½ lettuce and ½ brown rice + beans, tomatoes, steamed or grilled corn (no butter), and/or peppers

Platters

see above for sides

- ¼ Fire Grilled Chicken
- ½ Fire Grilled Chicken
- Boneless Chicken Breasts

Pollo Tropical (2)

Drink: Water

Family Meal

see above for sides

- Whole Fire-Grilled Chicken
  without rolls

Popeyes Louisiana Kitchen

Drink: Water

Sides

- Corn On The Cob
  without butter
- Red Beans
  without rice

Remember:
Many current diets make people think that eating healthily involves counting calories, limiting food consumption, complicated meal preparation, avoiding good protein sources, and/or eliminating carbs. Unfortunately, these common misconceptions about healthy eating lead some to adopt unrealistic and possibly harmful diets. These painful diets rely on dramatic changes of habits and often cause constant feelings of hunger and negative changes in mood.

Portillo's

Drink: Water

Sides

- Baked Potato (Plain)
  without: butter, cheese, bacon, sour cream, etc.
- Meatball
  without cheese
- Garden Side Salad
  without: cheese, croutons, and vinaigrette/dressing
- Fruit Cup

Salads

instead of dressing, ask for: lemon, pepper, vinegar, guacamole/avocados, or fresh salsa

- Chopped Salad
  without: pasta, bacon, cheese, and vinaigrette/dressing
- Caesar Salad (with Grilled Chicken Breast)
  without: Caesar dressing, croutons, and Parmesan cheese
- Greek Salad With Chicken
  without: cheese and vinaigrette/dressing
- Garden Side Salad
  without: cheese, croutons, and vinaigrette/dressing
- Tuscan Chicken Salad
  without: dressing, bacon, and walnuts (if candied, otherwise okay)

Chicken

- Char-Broiled Chicken Sandwich
  without: white bread (lettuce bun or whole wheat bun instead) and mayo

Portillo's (2)

Drink: Water

<u>Barnelli's Exclusives</u>

- Grilled Filet of Chicken
  without white bread (wheat and oat bran bun instead) and mayo
- Grilled Tuna Sandwich
  without white bread (wheat and oat bran bun instead) and tartar sauce

Remember:

Think results and after-effects... to say no to junk food now.

Thinking about how badly junk food makes the body feel can help stop you from eating junk food in the first place.

Potbelly Sandwich Shop

Drink: Water

Sandwiches

with multigrain or whole wheat bread
without white bread

- Turkey Breast
  without: cheese and mayo
- Mediterranean
  without: hummus and cheese
- Mediterranean Chicken
  without: hummus and cheese
- Smoked Ham
  without: cheese and mayo
- Roast Beef
  without: provolone cheese and mayo
- Clubby
  without: bacon, cheese, and ranch
- Vegetarian
  without: cheese and mayo

Salads

instead of dressing, ask for: lemon, pepper, vinegar, guacamole/avocados, or fresh salsa

- Powerhouse
  without: hummus and dressing
- Mediterranean
  without: cheese and dressing
- Uptown
  without: cheese, dried cranberries, candied walnuts, and dressing
- Farmhouse
  without: bacon, cheese, and dressing
- A Wreck Salad
  without: salami, cheese, and dressing

Potbelly Sandwich Shop (2)

Drink: Water

<u>Soups</u>

- Classic Tomato
- Garden Vegetable
- Homestyle Chicken Noodle
  without noodles

<u>Sides</u>

- Garden Side Salad
  without dressing

Remember:
Restaurant Survival Guide lists healthy food you can eat at restaurants to help you lose weight the simple way, without the pain of starvation or no-carb diets.

Qdoba

Drink: Water

Knockout Tacos

- Drunken Yardbird
  without: white flour tortilla (soft corn tortilla instead) and cheese
- Mad Rancher
  without: white flour tortilla (soft corn tortilla instead) bacon, ranch, and cheese
- Bohemian Veg
  without: white flour tortilla (soft corn tortilla instead) and cheese
- The Gladiator
  without: white flour tortilla (soft corn tortilla instead), bacon, and cheese

Burrito or Bowl

- Grilled Chicken or Steak
  with: wheat tortilla or bowl + brown rice + black beans + pico de gallo, roasted chile corn, salsa verde, and/or salsa roja + guacamole, shredded lettuce, and/or cilantro
  without: cheese and other sauce

Soup

- Tortilla Soup
  with only: chicken, guacamole, and cilantro. (without tortilla strips, cheese, and sour cream)

Red Lobster

Drink: Water

Soups & Salads

instead of dressing, ask for: lemon, pepper, vinegar, guacamole/avocados, or fresh salsa

- Classic Caesar Salad
  without: Parmesan, croutons, and dressing

Sides

- Asparagus
  without butter. steamed or grilled
- Baked Potato (Plain)
  without: butter, cheese, bacon, and sour cream
- Classic Caesar Salad
  without: Parmesan, croutons, and dressing
- Broccoli
  without butter. steamed or grilled
- Garden Salad
  without: cheese, croutons, and dressing

Shrimp

- Wood-Grilled Shrimp
  without butter
- Southwest-Style Tacos (Grilled Shrimp, Grilled Chicken, Fresh Tilapia)
  without: white flour tortillas (soft corn tortillas instead) and ranch
- Yucatán Tilapia and Shrimp
  without: butter, caramelized pineapple (grilled or fresh pineapple instead), and white rice (ask for side from above instead)

Shrimp

- Snow Crab Legs
  without butter

Red Lobster (2)

Drink: Water

Land & Sea

- Filet Mignon (6 oz.)
  without: butter and mashed potatoes (ask for side from above instead)
- 7 oz. Sirloin
  without: butter and mashed potatoes (ask for side from above instead)
- 12 oz. NY Strip
  without: butter and mashed potatoes (ask for side from above instead)
- Wood-Grilled Shrimp and Sirloin
  without: butter, caramelized pineapple (grilled or fresh pineapple instead), and white rice (ask for side from above instead)

Lobster & Signature Combos

- Wood-Grilled Lobster, Shrimp and Salmon
  without: butter and white rice (ask for side from above instead)
- Live Main Lobster
  see above for sides
- Rock Lobster Tails
  without: butter and white rice (ask for side from above instead)

Fish

- Canadian Walleye (Broiled)
  without: butter and white rice (ask for side from above instead)
- Wild-Caught Flounder (Broiled)
  without: butter and white rice (ask for side from above instead)

Red Robin Gourmet Burgers and Brews

Drink: Water

<u>Salads</u>

instead of dressing, ask for: lemon, pepper, vinegar, guacamole/avocados, or fresh salsa

- Avo-Cobb-O
  without: bacon, cheese, garlic toast, and dressing
- Simply Grilled Chicken Salad
  without: cheese, garlic toast, and dressing
- House Salad
  without: croutons, cheese, and dressing
- Southwest Salad
  without: fried jalapeño, cheese, and dressing
- Mighty Caesar Salad
  without: Parmesan, dressing, croutons, and garlic toast
- Side Caesar Salad
  without: Parmesan, dressing, croutons, and garlic toast

<u>Sides</u>

- Side Salad
  without: croutons, cheese, and dressing
- Steamed Broccoli
- Black Beans

<u>Other Fun On A Bun</u>

- Simply Grilled Chicken
  without: cheese, sauce, and white bread (ask for a whole wheat or lettuce bun instead)

Red Robin Gourmet Burgers and Brews (2)

Drink: Water

Gourmet Burgers

- Veggie Burger
  without: white bread bun (whole wheat/grain or lettuce bun instead), cheese, Parmesan-sprinkled mushrooms, and sauce

Entrées

- Ensenada Chicken
  without: cheese, tortilla strips, and ranch
- Sear-ious Salmon
  without coleslaw. ask for salmon to be cooked without butter and little to no oil

> Remember:
> With over 1,000 healthy menu options, this book helps busy folks like you to eat on the go, healthily, and without the pain that many other diets produce. It is an ongoing solution to promote long-term health.

Ruby Tuesday

Drink: Water

Salads

instead of dressing, ask for: lemon, pepper, vinegar, guacamole/avocados, or fresh salsa

- Endless Garden Bar
  without: dressing, cheese, dried cranberries, crispy onions, candied walnuts, crispy Parmesan chips, hummus, pasta salad, potato salad, ham & pea pasta, croutons, bacon, crackers, and olive oil

Soups

- Roasted Tomato
- Garden Vegetable

Burgers & Sandwiches

without white bread (whole wheat/grain or lettuce bun/bread instead)

- Triple Prime Burger
  without: sauce, mayo, cheese, and fries (garden bar instead)
- Avocado Turkey Burger
  without: bacon, sauce, mayo, cheese, and fries (garden bar instead)
- Grilled Chicken Sandwich
  without: sauce, mayo, cheese, and fries (garden bar instead)
- Avocado Grilled Chicken
  without: sauce, mayo, cheese, pickle chips, and fries (garden bar instead)

Chicken & Pasta

see below for sides

- Chicken Fresco
  without: lemon butter and balsamic vinaigrette
- Chicken 'Bella
  without: Parmesan cream sauce and lemon butter
  see below for sides

Ruby Tuesday (2)

Drink: Water

<u>Seafood & Steaks</u>

- Blackened Tilapia
  without butter. see below for sides
- Grilled Salmon
  without: sauce or butter. see below for sides
- Rib Eye
  without butter. see below for sides
- 6 oz. or 8 oz. Top Sirloin
  without butter. ask chef to cook with very little oil. see below for sides

<u>Sides</u>

- Garden Salad
  without: cheese, croutons, and dressing
- Steamed Broccoli
- Baked Potato (Plain)
  without: cheese, sour cream, and butter
- Grilled Zucchini
  without butter
- Sweet Potato (Plain)
  without: butter, sugar, marshmallows, candied walnuts, and jam

Ruth's Chris Steak House

Drink: Water

Steaks & Chops

ask for meat to be cooked without butter and with little to no oil

- Filet
- Cowboy Ribeye
- New York Strip
- Petite Filet & Shrimp
- Ribeye
- T-Bone
- Porterhouse For Two
- Petite Filet
- Petite Ribeye
- Lamb Chops
- Tomahawk Ribeye
- Bone-In Filet
- Bone-In New York Strip

Entrée Complements

- Shrimp
  without butter
- Lobster Tail
  without butter

Seafood & Specialties

- Chilean Sea Bass
  without butter. ask for sweet potato and pineapple hash to be cooked with little to no oil
- Vegetarian Plate
  without: cheese and butter. ask to be cooked with little to no oil

Ruth's Chris Steak House (2)

Drink: Water

<u>Appetizers & Sides</u>

- Roasted Brussel Sprouts
  without: butter and bacon. ask to be cooked with little to no oil
- Grilled Asparagus
  without: butter and sauce. ask to be cooked with little to no oil
- Fresh Broccoli
- Baked Potato (Plain)
  without: cheese, sour cream, bacon, and butter

<u>Soups & Salads</u>

instead of dressing, ask for: lemon, pepper, vinegar, guacamole/avocados, or fresh salsa

ask for meat to be cooked without butter and with little to no oil

- Steak House Salad
  without: croutons and dressing
- Ruth's Chop Salad
  without: bacon, cheese, dressing, and crispy onions
- Lettuce Wedge
  without: bacon, cheese, and dressing
- Harvest Salad
  without: bacon, dried cranberries, cheese, Cajun pecans, vinaigrette, and dressing
- Fresh Broccoli
- Baked Potato (Plain)
  without fixings (cheese, butter, sour cream, bacon, etc.)

Schlotzsky's

Drink: Water

Sandwiches

- Fresh Veggie
  without: cheese and dressing. with whole wheat/grain bread
- Smoked Turkey Breast
  without: sourdough (whole wheat/grain bread instead) and mayonnaise
- Fiesta Chicken Sandwich
  without: sourdough (whole wheat/grain bread instead), cheese, and chipotle mayo
- Turkey & Guacamole
  without: sauce or cheese. with whole wheat/grain bread
- Fiesta Chicken
  without: jalapeño cheese bun (whole wheat/grain bread instead), cheese, and chipotle mayo
- Angus Roast Beef
  without: sourdough bun (whole wheat/grain bread instead), cheese, pickles, mayo, and sauce

Soups

- Tomato Basil
  without cheese
- Garden Vegetable
  without: cheese, dried cranberries, candied pecans, croutons, garlic breadstick, and dressing
- Chicken Tortilla
  without: cheese and tortilla strips

Schlotzsky's (2)

Drink: Water

Salads

instead of dressing, ask for: lemon, pepper, vinegar, guacamole/avocados, or fresh salsa

- Fresh Kale & Grilled Chicken Salad
  without: cheese, dried cranberries, candied pecans, garlic breadstick, and dressing
- Cranberry, Apple, Pecan & Chicken Salad
  without: cheese, dried cranberries, candied pecans, croutons, garlic breadstick, and dressing
- Southwestern Chicken Salad
  without: cheese, tortilla strips, breadstick, and dressing
- Turkey Avocado Cobb Salad
  without: cheese, bacon, croutons, breadstick, and dressing
- Chicken Caesar Salad
  without: cheese, croutons, breadstick, and dressing

Remember:

While trendy diets and workout programs grow in popularity, the obesity rate is not decreasing. In fact, obesity related conditions like heart disease, stroke, type 2 diabetes and certain types of cancer continue to be some of the leading causes of preventable, premature death.

Helping restaurant-goers eat a sound meal is a need that was largely unmet by diet books… until now.

Sharky's

Drink: Water

Get It Naked

- Organic Roasted Vegetable Bowl
  without pesto (lemon, pico, or guacamole instead)
  Naked Chicken Fajita Bowl
  ask for fajitas to be cooked with little to no oil
- Naked Sharky's Chicken Salad
  without: dressing (lemon, pico, or guacamole instead)
- Wild Salmon "Lite" Burrito
  without aïoli
- Santa Fe "Lite" Burrito
  without cheese

Power Plates

with any of the following: organic poblano brown rice, organic quinoa with veggies, grilled veggies, organic black beans, organic pinto beans, steamed broccoli, organic Yucatan yams, organic roasted vegetables

- All Natural Chicken Breast
- All Natural Angus Steak
- Wild Caught Salmon
- Wild Caught Fish
- Shrimp

Tacos

with soft corn tortillas (without flour tortillas)

- Original
- California
  without cheese
- Organic Tofu & Veggies
- Wild Caught Fish or Shrimp
  without: cheese and sauce

Sharky's (2)

Drink: Water

Burritos

with low-fat whole wheat tortilla (without white flour tortilla)

- Fiesta (Chicken or Steak)
  without: white rice (brown rice instead), cheese, and sour cream (non-fat sour cream is okay)
- Sharky's (Chicken or Steak)
  without white rice (brown rice instead)
- Santa Fe (Chicken or Steak)
  without cheese
- Wild Caught Fish or Shrimp
  without: white rice (brown rice instead), cheese, and sauce
- Organic Tofu & Veggies

Salads

instead of dressing, ask for: lemon, pepper, vinegar, guacamole/avocados, or fresh salsa

optional add-ons: chicken, steak, wild caught salmon, grilled shrimp

- Summer Harvest
  without: dressing, raisins, and cheese
- Sharky's Chicken
  without: tortilla strips, rice noodles, and dressing
- Numex Caesar
  without: croutons, tortilla strips, cheese, and dressing
- Sharky's Quinoa
  without vinaigrette
- Side Salad
  without: croutons and cheese

Soup

- Chicken Tortilla
  without: tortilla strips, cheese, and sour cream (non-fat sour cream is okay)

Smashburger

Drink: Water

<u>Beef, Chicken, Turkey, or Black Bean Patty</u>

on a multigrain bun

ask for meat and bread not to be buttered

- Classic
  without: white bread bun, cheese, mayo, and sauce
- Avocado Club
  without: white bread bun, cheese, mayo, and sauce
- Spinach, Cucumber & Goat Cheese
  without: white bread bun, cheese, mayo, and sauce
- Create Your Own
  with: multigrain bun, avocado, grilled mushrooms, guacamole, cucumbers, spinach, lettuce, tomatoes, and onion
  without: white bread bun, sauce and dressing, cheese, and fries

<u>Salads</u>

instead of dressing, ask for: lemon, pepper, vinegar, guacamole/avocados, or fresh salsa

- Classic Cobb Salad
  without: bacon, cheese, ranch, and dressing
- Spinach, Cucumber & Goat Cheese Salad
  without: cheese, vinaigrette, and dressing

Sonic

Drink: Water

Chicken

- Classic Grilled Chicken
  without: white bread (lettuce bun instead), cheese, mayo, sauce, and fries

Steak 'n Shake

Drink: Water

Specialty Steakburgers

- Fresh Guacamole
  without: white bread (lettuce bun instead), cheese, mayo, sauce, and fries

Specialty Sandwiches

- Grilled Chicken Sandwich
  without: white bread (lettuce bun instead), cheese, mayo, sauce, and fries

Salads

- Fresh Guacamole
  without: cheese, croutons, and dressing
- Grilled Chicken Salad
  without: cheese, croutons, and dressing

Subway

Drink: Water

<u>Sandwiches & Flatbreads</u>

with 9-Grain Wheat, Multigrain Flatbread, or Rye
+ veggies
+ (optional) guacamole
+ (optional) red wine vinegar
without cheese, bacon, pepperoni, sauce, and dressing

- Oven Roasted Chicken
- Black Forest Ham
- Roast Beef
- Rotisserie-Style Chicken
- Turkey Breast
- Veggie Delite

<u>Salads</u>

+ veggies
+ (optional) guacamole
+ (optional) red wine vinegar
without cheese, bacon, pepperoni, sauce, and dressing

- Oven Roasted Chicken
- Black Forest Ham
- Roast Beef
- Rotisserie-Style Chicken
- Turkey Breast
- Veggie Delite

Taco Bell

Drink: Water

<u>Power Menu</u>

instead of dressing, ask for: lemon, pepper, vinegar, guacamole/avocados, or fresh salsa

- Power Bowl (Chicken)
  without: cheese, rice, ranch, sauce, dressing, and sour cream
  (optional add-ons) only: lettuce, onions, tomatoes, and beans
- Power Bowl (Veggie)
  without: cheese, rice, ranch, sauce, dressing, and sour cream
  (optional add-ons) only: lettuce, onions, tomatoes, and beans

<u>Sides</u>

- Black Beans
  (optional add-ons and upgrades) only: chicken, lettuce, onions, tomatoes, beans, guacamole, and onions

Remember:
Restaurant Survival Guide is intended to help users lose body fat. To help you sculpt abs and other muscles, we recommend the Ocinator Fitness Program as the ideal companion to this book. Ocinator workouts are simple and do not aim for sweat and exhaustion. On the contrary, Ocinator workouts were designed to minimize workout time (20 minutes/day) and pain so that users can realistically maintain results and a positive long-term change in fitness lifestyle.

Taco Cabana

Drink: Water

Breakfast

- Egg Taco
  without: flour tortilla (soft corn tortilla instead), cheese, bacon, and chorizo

Tacos

- Flame-Grilled USDA Choice Steak Street Tacos
  with soft corn tortilla
- Shredded Chicken Taco
  without: flour tortilla (soft corn tortilla instead) and cheese
- Black Bean Taco
  without: flour tortilla (soft corn tortilla instead) and rice

Bowls

- Bowl with No Shell (Grilled Chicken or Steak)
  without: rice, sour cream, and cheese

Sides

- Refried Beans
  without cheese
- Black Beans
  without cheese
- Guacamole

Taco John's

Drink: Water

<u>Tacos</u>

- Street Tacos (Sirloin steak or Grilled Chicken
  without: flour tortillas (soft corn tortillas instead), garlic lime sauce, and cheese. if soft corn tortillas are not available, ask for more lettuce as a substitute

<u>Sides</u>

instead of dressing, ask for: lemon, pepper, vinegar, guacamole/avocados, or fresh salsa

- Refried Beans
  without cheese
- Side Salad
  without: cheese and dressing

Remember:
Both *Restaurant Survival Guide* and Ocinator Fitness aim to make obtaining and maintaining long-term fitness results simple and realistic.
See Ocinator.com for more details.
Now… it's time to enjoy all your new restaurant menu options <u>and</u> feel great!

Texas de Brazil Churrascaria

Drink: Water

Meats

don't eat the meat fat

- Pinanha
- Leg of Lamb
- Lamb Chops
- Garlic Picanha
- Filet Mignon
- Flank Steak

Salad Area

without dressing and vinaigrette. instead, ask for: lemon, pepper, vinegar, guacamole/avocados, or fresh salsa

- Tomato Slices
- Steamed Asparagus
- Malgueta Peppers
- Heart of Palm
- Romaine Lettuce
- Ceviche Onions
- Roasted Red & Yellow Peppers
- Tabbouleh
- Couscous Salad
- Marinated Artichoke Hearts
- Roasted Jalapeños
- Sushi (brown rice)
  without white rice
- Smoked Salmon
- Peppadew Peppers
- Pepperoncini
- Sun-Dried Cherry Tomatoes
- Kalamata Olives
- Cherry Tomatoes

Hot Items

- Moqueca Fish Stew
- Brazilian Black Beans (if cooked without bacon)

Texas Roadhouse

Drink: Water

Salads

instead of dressing, ask for: lemon, pepper, vinegar, guacamole/avocados, or fresh salsa

- Grilled Chicken Salad
  without: cheese, bacon, croutons, and dressing
- Steakhouse Filet Salad
  without: cheese, bacon, croutons, and dressing. ask for steak to be cooked without butter and with little to no oil
- House Salad
  without: cheese, croutons, and dressing
- Caesar Salad
  without: cheese, croutons, and dressing
- Chicken Caesar Salad
  without: cheese, croutons, and dressing

Sides

- Fresh Vegetables
  without butter
- House Salad
  without: cheese, croutons, and dressing
- Caesar Salad
  without: cheese, croutons, and dressing
- Baked Potato (Plain)
  without: cheese, bacon, butter, sour cream, etc.
- Sweet Potato (Plain)
  without: marshmallows and caramel sauce
- Green Beans (Steamed)
  without: butter and oil

Country Dinners

- Country Vegetable Plate
  see above for sides

Texas Roadhouse (2)

Drink: Water

Chicken Specialties

see above for sides

- Oven Roasted Half Chicken
  without: cheese, bacon, croutons, and dressing

Steaks

ask for steak to be cooked without butter and with little to no oil
see above for sides

- Ft. Worth Ribeye
- Dallas Filet
- USDA Choice Sirloin
- New York Strip
- Porterhouse T-Bone
- Steak Kabob
  without white rice

Dockside Favorites

see above for sides

- Grilled Shrimp
  without: butter and white rice (ask for fresh vegetables instead). ask for shrimp to be cooked with little to no oil
- Grilled Salmon
  without butter. ask for salmon to be cooked with little to no oil

Burgers & Sandwiches

see above for sides

- Chicken Sandwich
  without: white bread bun (whole wheat/grain or lettuce bun instead) sautéed mushrooms (grilled instead), and cheese
- Burger
  without: white bread bun (whole wheat/grain or lettuce bun instead), bacon, sautéed mushrooms (grilled instead), and cheese

TGI Fridays

Drink: Water

Sides

- House Salad
  without: cheese, croutons, and dressing
- Caesar Salad
  without: cheese, croutons, Parmesan crisps, and dressing
- Super Veggies

Salads & Soups

instead of dressing, ask for: lemon, pepper, vinegar, guacamole/avocados, and/or fresh salsa

- House Salad
  without: cheese, croutons, dressing, and breadstick
- Caesar Salad
  without: cheese, croutons, Parmesan crisps, dressing, and breadstick
- Strawberry Fields Salad With Grilled Chicken
  without: cheese, Parmesan, glazed pecans, dressing/vinaigrette, and breadstick
- Caesar Salad With Grilled Chicken
  without: cheese, croutons, Parmesan crisps, dressing, and breadstick
- Million Dollar Cobb
  without: bacon, cheese, Parmesan, dressing, vinaigrette/dressing, and breadstick

Appetizers

- Grilled Wings
  without: sauce and dressing

TGI Fridays (2)

Drink: Water

Burgers

see above for sides

- Turkey Burger
  without: white bread (lettuce or whole wheat bun instead), sauce, and fries
- Burger
  without: white bread bun (whole wheat/grain or lettuce bun instead), bacon, sautéed mushrooms (grilled instead), and cheese

Sandwiches

see above for sides

- Turkey + Avocado
  without: white bread (lettuce or whole wheat bun instead), bacon, Swiss, sauce, pesto, and fries

Chicken, Seafood & Pasta

see above for sides

- Dragon-Glaze Salmon
  without: glaze and white rice (brown rice or more veggies instead)
- Dragon-Glaze Chicken
  without: glaze and white rice (brown rice or more veggies instead)

Steaks & Ribs

don't eat the meat fat

- Center-Cut Sirloin
  without: butter and mashed potatoes (brown rice or more veggies instead)
- New York Strip
  without: butter and mashed potatoes (brown rice or more veggies instead)

The Capital Grille

Drink: Water

Salads

instead of dressing, ask for: lemon, pepper, vinegar, guacamole/avocados, and/or fresh salsa

- Maine Lobster Salad
  without: vinaigrette/dressing
- Caesar Salad With All-Natural Chicken Breast
  without: cheese, croutons, Parmesan crisps, and dressing
- Seared Salmon With Avocado, Mango, and Tomato Salad
  without: champagne vinaigrette/dressing
- The Capital Grille "Cobb" Salad With Sliced Tenderloin
  without vinaigrette/dressing
- Seared Tuna Salad
  ask for tuna to be cooked with little no oil
  without vinaigrette/dressing

Burgers and Sandwiches

without Parmesan truffle fries or chips. see above for sides to ask for instead

- Lobster and Crab Burger
  without: white bread bun (ask for whole wheat/grain bun or lettuce bun instead) and tartar sauce
- Ribeye Steak Sandwich
  without: white bread bun (ask for whole wheat/grain bun or lettuce bun instead), sauce, caramelized onions (grilled onions instead), and Havarti
- Maine Lobster Roll
  without: brioche bun (ask for whole wheat/grain bun or lettuce bun instead), tartar sauce, bacon, and cheese

The Capital Grille (2)

Drink: Water

Plates

with field greens salad, no croutons, cheese, dressing and vinaigrette instead of dressing, ask for: lemon, pepper, vinegar, guacamole/avocados, and/or fresh salsa

- Seared Salmon with Asparagus and Shiitakes
  ask for salmon, asparagus, and shiitakes to be cooked with little to no oil
  without parsnip purée
- Mini Tenderloin Sandwiches
  without: white bread bun (ask for whole wheat/grain bun or lettuce bun instead), sauce, caramelized onions (grilled onions instead), cheese, and Parmesan truffle fries
- Grilled Breast of Chicken
  without: caramelized onions (grilled onions instead)
  ask for baby potatoes to be cooked without oil

Entrées

with steamed or grilled green beans (not French) or a salad without cheese, croutons, and dressing/vinaigrette

- Filet Mignon 8 oz
- Bone-In Dry Aged NY Strip
  without: cheese, croutons, Parmesan crisps, and dressing
- Sushi-Grade Sesame Seared Tuna
  ask for tuna to be cooked with little to no oil
  without: white rice (ask more green beans or salad instead) and sauces
- Roasted Swordfish
  without gratin (ask more green beans or salad instead)
- Sliced Filet Mignon
  without cipollini mushrooms. ask for vegetables to be cooked with little to no oil

The Cheesecake Factory

Drink: Water

Appetizer Salads

- Tossed Green Salad
  without: croutons and vinaigrette/dressing
- French Country Salad
  without: goat cheese, candied pecans, and vinaigrette/dressing
- Fresh Vegetable Salad
  without: cheese and vinaigrette/dressing
- Factory Chopped Salad
  without: bacon, cheese, and vinaigrette/dressing

Salads

instead of dressing, ask for: lemon, pepper, vinegar, guacamole/avocados, and/or fresh salsa

- Caesar Salad
  without: croutons, cheese, and dressing
- Sheila's Chicken and Avocado Salad
  without: tortilla strips and vinaigrette/dressing
- Chinese Chicken Salad
  without: white rice noodles, crisp wontons, and vinaigrette/dressing
- Chicken, Mango, and Avocado Salad
  without: crispy wontons and vinaigrette/dressing
- Chipotle Grilled Shrimp Salad
  without: cheese and vinaigrette/dressing
- Santa Fe Salad
  without: cheese, tortilla strips, and vinaigrette/dressing
- Cobb Salad
  without: bacon, cheese, and vinaigrette/dressing
- Seared Tuna Tataki Salad
  without vinaigrette/dressing

The Cheesecake Factory (2)

Drink: Water

Appetizers

- Fire-Roasted Fresh Artichoke
  without garlic dip
- Guacamole
  without tortilla chips (ask for soft corn tortillas instead if available)

Small Plates & Snacks

- Little House Salad
  without vinaigrette/dressing
- Greek Salad
  without: cheese and vinaigrette/dressing
- Edamame
  without gratin (ask more green beans or salad instead)

"Super" Foods

- Avocado Toast (if whole grain/wheat bread is available)
  without: white bread (ask for whole wheat/grain bread instead) and olive oil
- California Guacamole Salad
  without: crispy tortillas, feta cheese, and dressing/vinaigrette (guacamole is okay)
- Wellness Salad
  without: roasted pear, sunflower seeds, and vinaigrette/dressing
- Kale and Quinoa Salad
  without: Parmesan cheese, sunflower seeds, and vinaigrette/dressing
- Vegan Cobb Salad
  without: sunflower seeds and vinaigrette/dressing
- Almond-Crusted Salmon Salad
  ask for salmon to be cooked with little to no oil
  without: dried cranberries and vinaigrette/dressing

The Cheesecake Factory (3)

Drink: Water

<u>Glamburgers & Sandwiches</u>

without fries. instead, ask for green salad without dressing, croutons, and cheese

- Grilled Turkey Burger
  without sauce/dressing
- Veggie Burger
  without: cheese, garlic aïoli, and sauce/dressing
- Grilled Chicken And Avocado Club
  without: white bread (whole wheat/grain or lettuce bun instead), Swiss, mayo, and fries
- Southwest Chicken Sandwich
  without: white bread (whole wheat/grain or lettuce bun instead) and chipotle mayo
- Impossible Burger
  without: white bread (whole wheat/grain or lettuce bun instead) and sauce

<u>Specialties</u>

- Chicken Enchiladas
  without: cheese (on enchiladas and beans) and cilantro rice (more corn without butter instead)
- Baja Chicken Tacos
  without: cheese (in tacos and on beans) and cilantro rice (more corn without butter instead)
- Baja Chicken Tacos
  without: cheese (in tacos and on beans) and cilantro rice (more corn without butter instead)

The Cheesecake Factory (4)

Drink: Water

<u>Steaks, Chops, Fish & Seafood</u>

without butter and little to no oil

- Carne Asada
  without: sauce, white rice (ask for more corn without butter and cheese instead), sautéed vegetables (ask for grilled vegetables with little to no oil instead), and butter and cheese (on corn)
- Chargrilled Bone-In New York Steak
  without mashed potatoes (more vegetables instead)
- Grilled Rib-Eye Steak
  without mashed potatoes (more vegetables instead)
- Filet Mignon
  without mashed potatoes (more vegetables instead)
- Fresh Grilled Salmon
  without: sauce and mashed potatoes (more broccoli/vegetables instead)
- Herb Crusted Filet of Salmon
  without: lemon sauces and mashed potatoes (more asparagus/vegetables instead)

<u>Skinnylicious Small Plates and Appetizers</u>

- Greek Salad
  without: feta cheese and vinaigrette/dressing
- Little House Salad
  without vinaigrette/dressing
- Skinnylicious Grilled Artichoke
  without lemon-garlic aïoli
- Chicken Lettuce Wrap Tacos (Asian or Mexican)
  without: white rice noodles and sauce/dressing on chicken
- Ahi Tartare
  without soy-ginger sesame sauce

The Cheesecake Factory (5)

Drink: Water

Skinnylicious Salads

instead of dressing, ask for: lemon, pepper, vinegar, guacamole/avocados, and/or fresh salsa

- Skinnylicious Tossed Green Salad
  without: croutons and dressing
- Skinnylicious French Country Salad
  without: goat cheese, candied pecans, and vinaigrette/dressing
- Skinnylicious Caesar Salad
  without: croutons, cheese, and dressing
- Skinnylicious Fresh Vegetable Salad
  without: cheese and vinaigrette/dressing
- Skinnylicious Factory Chopped Salad
  without: bacon, cheese, and vinaigrette/dressing
- Skinnylicious Asian Chicken Salad
  without: white rice noodles, crisp wontons, and vinaigrette/dressing
- Skinnylicious Mexican Tortilla Salad
  without: crispy corn tortilla (soft corn tortillas instead), cheese, tortilla strips, avocado cream sauce (plain avocados instead), sour cream, and vinaigrette/dressing
- Skinnylicious Seared Tuna Tataki Salad
  ask for tuna to be seared with little to no oil
  without wasabi vinaigrette

The Cheesecake Factory (6)

Drink: Water

<u>Skinnylicious Specialties</u>

without fries. ask for green salad without dressing, croutons, and cheese instead

- Skinnylicious Hamburger
  without: white bread bun (whole wheat/grain or lettuce bun instead), pickles, and mayonnaise
- Skinnylicious Veggie Burger
  without: white bread bun (whole wheat/grain or lettuce bun instead), pickles, and mayonnaise
- Skinnylicious Grilled Turkey Burger
  without: white bread bun (whole wheat/grain or lettuce bun instead) and mayonnaise
- Skinnylicious Turkey & Avocado Sandwich
  without: white bread bun (whole wheat/grain or lettuce bun instead), bacon, and mayonnaise
- Skinnylicious Soft Tacos
  without: crema and escabeche vegetables (grilled or steamed vegetables instead)
- Skinnylicious Chicken Enchiladas
  without: cheese and escabeche vegetables (grilled or steamed vegetables instead)
- Skinnylicious Tuscan Chicken
  without: balsamic vinaigrette and sauce
- Skinnylicious Grilled Salmon
  without: balsamic vinaigrette and sauce

The Cheesecake Factory (7)

Drink: Water

<u>Eggs & Omelettes</u>

ask for eggs to be cooked without butter and with little to no oil

- Farm Fresh Eggs
  with: tomatoes or whole wheat/grain toast
- Factory Huevos Rancheros
  without: cheese (on eggs and beans), crispy tortillas (soft corn tortillas instead), and sour cream
- Factory Create An Omelette
  with four of the following: ham, avocado, peppers, mushrooms, asparagus, spinach, bell peppers, tomato, red or green onions
- California Omelette
  without cheese (in tacos and on beans), chorizo, and sour cream
- Spinach and Mushroom Omelette
  without: cheese (in tacos and on beans), sautéed mushrooms (grilled instead), bacon, and sour cream
- Breakfast Tacos
  without: cheese (in tacos and on beans), and sour cream

Remember:

Small changes make a huge difference.

It might seem like the difference between white bread and whole grain bread, water and lemonade, dressing and no dressing, are of little significance. False. These small changes are what allow you to lose fat without spending all day doing cardio.

The Habit Burger Grill

Drink: Water

Charburgers

without fries

- Charburger
  without: white bread bun (whole wheat bun instead), caramelized onions, pickles, and sauce/dressing
- Double Charburger
  without: white bread bun (whole wheat bun instead), caramelized onions, pickles, mayo, and sauce/dressing
- Santa Barbara Char
  without: white bread bun (whole wheat bun instead), cheese, caramelized onions, pickles, and sauce/dressing

Salads

instead of dressing, ask for: lemon, pepper, vinegar, guacamole/avocados, and/or fresh salsa

- Garden Salad
  without: croutons, cheese, and dressing/vinaigrette
- Grilled Chicken Salad
  without: croutons, cheese, and dressing/vinaigrette
- Grilled Chicken Caesar
  without: Caesar dressing, croutons, cheese, and dressing/vinaigrette
- Super Food Salad
  without: Craisins, cheese, and dressing/vinaigrette
- Santa Barbara Cobb
  without: bacon, cheese, croutons, and dressing/vinaigrette
- Caesar Salad
  without: Caesar dressing, croutons, cheese, and dressing/vinaigrette

The Habit Burger Grill (2)

Drink: Water

Sandwiches

instead of dressing, ask for: lemon, pepper, vinegar, guacamole/avocados, and/or fresh salsa

- Veggie Burger
  without sweet mustard

Sides

- Side Caesar Salad
  without: Caesar dressing, croutons, cheese, and dressing/vinaigrette
- Side Salad
  without: cheese (on eggs and beans), crispy tortillas (soft corn tortillas instead), and sour cream

Tim Hortons

Drink: Water

Sandwiches

without white bread bun (lettuce bun instead), bacon, cheese, and sauce/dressing

- Turkey
- Ham

Soups

- Hearty Vegetable
- Chicken Noodle
  without noodles

Breakfast

- Homestyle Oatmeal (Mixed Berries or Plain)
  without added sugar

Tropical Smoothie Cafe

Drink: Water

<u>Bowls</u>

- Baja Chicken Bowl
  without: pickled red onion, cheese, and dressing/vinaigrette
- Supergreen Caesar Chicken Bowl
  without: Parmesan, Parmesan crisps, and Caesar dressing
- Santa Barbara Char
  without: white bun (whole wheat or lettuce bun instead), cheese, caramelized onions, pickles, and sauce/dressing

<u>Superfood Smoothies</u>

without any added sugar

- Acai Berry Boost
- Avocolada
- Chia Banana Boost
  without peanut butter
- Chia Banana Max
  without peanut butter
- Detox Island Green
  without natural sweetener
- Health Nut
- Acai Island Green
- Lean Machine
- Muscle Blaster
- Orange Ginger Glow
- Pomegranate Plunge
- Triple Berry Oat
  without Splenda

Tropical Smoothie Café (2)

Drink: Water

Classic Smoothies

without any added sugar or juice (fruit only)

- Blueberry Bliss
- Jetty Punch
- Kiwi Quencher
  without peanut butter
- Mango Magic
  without peanut butter
- Paradise Point
  without natural sweetener
- Peaches 'N Silk
- Strawberry Limeade

Sandwiches

without fries. ask for green salad without dressing, croutons, and cheese instead

- Turkey
  with: 9-grain bread, lettuce, and tomatoes
  without: bacon, cheese, and honey dijon

Village Inn

Drink: Water

<u>Dinner</u>

- Lemon Artichoke Chicken
  without: white rice, lemon-parsley butter sauce, and sautéed spinach (ask for grilled spinach without oil instead)
  ask for an extra side from below instead
- Top Sirloin
  without: butter, mashed potatoes, and gravy
  (ask for two other sides from below instead)
- Slow Roasted Turkey
  without: stuffing, mashed potatoes, and gravy
  (ask for two other sides from below instead)

<u>Lunch</u>

with fresh fruit, side salad (see Sides details below), or tomato basil soup

- Turkey Avocado Sandwich
  without: bacon, cheese, and mayo
- Burger
  without: white bread bun (wheat bread bun or lettuce bun instead), cheese, bacon, onion rings, and dressing
  with: tomato, lettuce, fresh onions
- All-White Meat Chicken Breast Burger
  without: white bread bun (wheat bread bun or lettuce bun instead), cheese, bacon, onion rings, and dressing
  with: tomato, lettuce, fresh onions
- Classy Cobb Salad
  without: bacon, cheese, and dressing/vinaigrette
- Celebrity Chef Salad
  without: cheese, croutons, and dressing/vinaigrette
- Southwest Salad
  without: crispy tortilla strips and dressing/vinaigrette

Village Inn (2)

Drink: Water or Low-Fat Milk

<u>Sides</u>

instead of dressing, ask for: lemon, pepper, vinegar, guacamole/avocados, and/or fresh salsa

- Tomato Basil Soup
- Side Garden Salad
  without: cheese, croutons, dressing, and dressing/vinaigrette
- Fresh Fruit
- Fresh Broccoli
- Green Beans
  without butter
- Corn
  without butter

<u>Breakfast</u>

ask for eggs to be cooked without butter and with little to no oil

- Top Sirloin & Eggs
  ask for eggs and sirloin to be cooked without butter
  without: pancakes and hash browns
- California Skillet
  ask for skillet to be cooked with little to no oil
  without: bacon, cheese, and hollandaise. (ask for potatoes to be cooked without oil and ask for eggs to be cooked without butter)

Village Inn (3)

Drink: Water or Low-Fat Milk

Omelettes

without buttermilk pancakes and hash browns. multigrain pancakes (ask to be cooked with little to no sugar) instead

- Denver Omelette
  without cheese
- Fresh Spinach & Bacon Omelette
  without: bacon, cheese, and hollandaise sauce
- Garden Veggie Omelette
  without cheese
- Create Your Own Omelette
  without cheese
  with any of the following: onions, mushrooms, fresh spinach, tomatoes, broccoli, green peppers, artichokes, ham, and avocado
- Tres Huevos Rancheros
  without: cheese (on eggs and beans), crispy corn tortillas (soft corn tortillas instead), pork green chili, and sour cream
- Fruit & Nut Multigrain Pancakes
  ask to be cooked with little to no sugar
  without: jam, jelly, preserves, and syrup

Breakfast Sides

- Fresh Fruit
- Cinnamon Apples
  without added sugar
- Quaker Oatmeal (plain)
  without added sugar
- Whole Grain/Wheat Toast (if available)

Waffle House

Drink: Water or Low-Fat Milk

Breakfast

- ask for eggs cooked without butter and with little to no oil and only get toast if whole wheat/grain bread is available

Toddle House Omelettes

- Ham
  without cheese
- Fiesta
  without cheese

Steak & Eggs

- T-Bone & Eggs
  without cheese
- Steak & Eggs
  without: bacon, cheese, and hollandaise sauce
- Grilled Chicken& Eggs
  without cheese

Eggs

ask for eggs to be cooked without butter and with little to no oil

- 3 Eggs
- 2 Eggs
- 1 Egg

Waffle House (2)

Drink: Water or Low-Fat Milk

Lunch & Dinner

garden salad without croutons, cheese, and dressing, without hash browns and white bread toast (get whole wheat/grain bread without butter if available). ask for more salad instead

- T-Bone Steak
- Sirloin
- Grilled Chicken
  without cheese
- Grilled Chicken Sandwich
  without: white bread bun (whole wheat/grain bun or lettuce bun instead), cheese, bacon, and sauce/dressing

We hope this book will help you enjoy eating out at the most popular U.S. chain restaurants. And that the food recommendations within will help you look and feel as fit and fantastic as you deserve to be.

Wendy's

Drink: Water

Chicken

- Grilled Chicken Sandwich
  without: white bread (whole wheat/grain bun or lettuce bun instead), honey mustard, and cheese

Fresh-Made Salads

instead of dressing, ask for: lemon, pepper, vinegar, guacamole/avocados, and/or fresh salsa

- Harvest Salad
  without: cheese, dried cranberries, brown sugar walnuts, bacon, and dressing/vinaigrette
- Southwest Avocado Chicken Salad
  without: bacon, cheese, ranch, and dressing/vinaigrette
- Apple Pecan Chicken Salad
  without: cheese, cranberries, roasted pecans (if sweetened), and dressing/vinaigrette
- Chicken Caesar Salad
  ask for grilled, not crispy chicken
  without: crispy chicken, cheese, croutons, and dressing/vinaigrette

Sides

- Plain Baked Potato
  without: cheese, dried cranberries, brown sugar walnuts, bacon, and dressing/vinaigrette
- Side Caesar Salad
  without: cheese, croutons, and dressing/vinaigrette
- Apple Bites

Breakfast

- Apple Bites

Whataburger

Drink: Water

Chicken

- Grilled Chicken Sandwich
  without: white bread (whole wheat/grain or lettuce bun instead), sauce, and cheese

Burgers

without cheese, mustard, and white bread (whole wheat/grain or lettuce bun instead)

- Whataburger
- Double Meat Whataburger

Sides

instead of dressing, ask for: lemon, pepper, vinegar, guacamole/avocados, and/or fresh salsa

- Apple Chicken Salad (with Grilled Chicken)
  without: cheese, cranberries, and dressing/vinaigrette
- Garden Salad
  without: cheese, croutons, and dressing/vinaigrette
- Apple Bites

Remember:

There's no need to eliminate carbs, starve yourself, have a rigorous meal plan, or count calories! You can have the strength, energy, and positivity provided by delicious healthy food and be fit! The latest medical research shows that losing weight is as simple as not eating products with added sugar and refined grain. We also need lots of vegetables.

Yard House

Drink: Water

Snacks

- Guacamole
  without: chips (ask for soft corn tortillas instead) and feta
- Chilled Edamame
- Street Tacos A La Carte (Baja Fish, Baja Shrimp, Blackened Shrimp, Asada, or Chipotle Chicken)
  without: flour tortillas (soft corn tortillas instead), cheese, and sauce (salsa is okay)
- Ahi Sashimi
  without soy vinaigrette
- Chicken Lettuce Wraps
  without sauce
- Spicy Tuna Roll (if brown rice is available)
  without: white rice (brown rice instead) and soy sauce

Starter Soups & Salads

instead of dressing, ask for: lemon, pepper, vinegar, guacamole/avocados, and/or fresh salsa

- Tomato Bisque
  without: cheese, dried cranberries, and dressing/vinaigrette
- Traditional Caesar
  without: Parmesan crisps, croutons, and Caesar dressing
- Kale Caesar
  without: raisins, Parmesan crisps, croutons, and Caesar dressing
- Chopped Salad
  without: bacon and dressing/vinaigrette
- Mixed Field Greens
  without: croutons and dressing/vinaigrette

Yard House (2)

Drink: Water or Low-Fat Milk

<u>Entrée Salads</u>

instead of dressing, ask for: lemon, pepper, vinegar, guacamole/avocados, and/or fresh salsa

- Chicken Kale Caesar (Chicken, Shrimp, Skirt Steak, Salmon, or Ahi)
  without: raisins, Parmesan crisps, croutons, and Caesar dressing
- Cobb Salad (Chicken, Shrimp, Skirt Steak, or Salmon)
  without: cheese, bacon, and dressing/vinaigrette
- Red Quinoa Salad
  without: cheese and dressing/vinaigrette

<u>House Favorites</u>

- Chicken Enchilada Stack
  without: cheese, sour cream, and rice (more beans without cheese or brown rice instead)
- Poke Bowl
  without: crispy rice, crispy wonton, soy vinaigrette, and sriracha aïoli

<u>Steaks</u>

- Rib Eye
  without: butter, mashed potatoes (plain baked potato instead), broccoli (fresh or grilled vegetables without dressing instead), and steak sauce
- Skirt Steak Arrachera
  without: butter (on steak and corn) and white rice (brown rice or beans without cheese instead)
- Rib Eye & Shrimp
  without: butter, steak sauce, mashed potatoes (plain baked potato instead), and broccoli (fresh or grilled vegetables without dressing instead)

Yard House (3)

Drink: Water

<u>Seafood</u>

- Pan Seared Ahi
  ask for Ahi to be seared with little to no oil
  without: sauce and white rice (brown rice or more vegetables instead)
- Mediterranean Salmon
  without: tahini and raisins
- Ginger Crusted Salmon
  without: butter, peanut vinaigrette, and mashed potatoes (plain baked potato instead)

<u>Street Tacos</u>

with soft corn tortillas, not flour tortillas

- Baja Shrimp or Baja Fish
  without sriracha aïoli
- Blackened Shrimp
  without cumin crema
- Asada
- Chipotle Chicken
  without: sauce, cheese, and cumin crema

<u>Burgers</u>

without white bread bun (lettuce, whole wheat/grain, or rye bun instead)

- Beef Burger
  without: cheese, sauce, aïoli, and fries (vegetables instead)
- Turkey Burger
  without: cheese, aïoli, and fries (vegetables instead)
- Vegan Burger
  without: onion bun, sauce, and cheese
- Lamb Burger
  without: sauce, cheese, caramelized jalapeño shallot relish, and fries (vegetables instead)

Yard House (4)

Drink: Water

<u>Sandwiches</u>

without white bread. ask for lettuce bun, whole wheat/grain bun, or rye bun instead

- Grilled Chicken & Avocado Sandwich
  without: cheese, mayo, and fries (vegetables instead)
- Roasted Turkey Club
  without: cheese, bacon, mayo, sourdough, and fries (vegetables instead)
- Seared Ahi Steak Sandwich
  ask for Ahi to be seared with little to no oil
  without: cheese, caramelized onions (grilled onions instead), aïoli, and fries (vegetables instead)

> Remember:
> It's common sense that a calorie is not just a calorie. We should be eating lots of good calories and few bad calories! For example, eating 500 calories of vegetables is much healthier than eating 100 calories of a donut.

Zaxby's

- Drink: Water

<u>Zalads</u>

instead of dressing, ask for: lemon, pepper, vinegar, guacamole/avocados, and/or fresh salsa

- The House (Grilled Chicken)
  without: cheese, fried onions, dressing/vinaigrette, and white bread toast (whole wheat/grain toast instead, if available)
- The Cobb (Grilled Chicken)
  without: cheese, bacon, fried onions, dressing/vinaigrette, and white bread toast (whole wheat/grain toast instead, if available)
- The Caesar
  without: cheese, bacon, croutons, dressing/vinaigrette, and white bread toast (whole wheat/grain toast instead, if available)

<u>Sides & Extras</u>

- Basket of Celery
  without dressing/sauce
- Side Salad
  without: cheese, croutons, and dressing/vinaigrette

> Remember:
> Carry this book with you to help you choose a restaurant, order, and eat out healthily.

Zoës Kitchen

Drink: Water

Starters

- Mediterranean Lamb Kafta
  without: tzatziki and harissa

Soups & Salads

instead of dressing, ask for: lemon, pepper, vinegar, guacamole/avocados, and/or fresh salsa

- Chicken & Orzo Soup
  without orzo
- Mediterranean Lentil Soup
  without: cheese, croutons, and dressing/vinaigrette
- Live Med Salad
  without: Parmesan cheese and dressing/vinaigrette
- Quinoa Salad
  without: feta and dressing/vinaigrette
- Greek Salad
  without: feta, potato salad, and pita bread
- Tossed Greek Salad
  without: pasta salad, caramelized onions (grilled onions instead), feta, dressing/vinaigrette, and pita

Sandwiches

- Turkey Stack
  without: sourdough (7-grain or rye bread instead), feta spread, and rosemary oil
- Steak Stack
  without: sourdough (7-grain or rye bread instead), feta spread, and rosemary oil

Zoës Kitchen (2)

Drink: Water

Kabobs

- Chicken Kabobs
  without: feta, oil, and dressing/vinaigrette on salad
- Steak Kabobs
  without: Italian salsa verde and feta, oil, and dressing/vinaigrette on salad
- Salmon Kabobs
  without: Moroccan harissa and feta, oil, and dressing/vinaigrette on salad
- Shrimp Kabobs
  without: tzatziki and feta, oil, and dressing/vinaigrette on salad

Bowls & Classics

- Cauliflower Rice Bowl
  without: feta, tzatziki, Israeli skhug, oil, and dressing/vinaigrette
- Power Grain Bowl
  without: tzatziki, Moroccan harissa, Mediterranean relish, oil, and dressing/vinaigrette
- Mediterranean Salad Trio Bowl
  without: pesto farro (plain farro instead), tzatziki, Italian salsa verde, feta, oil, and dressing/vinaigrette
- Mediterranean Chicken
  without: caramelized onions and feta, oil, and dressing/vinaigrette on salad

Zoës Kitchen (3)

Drink: Water

Family Dinners

- Moroccan Chicken Family Dinner
  without: white rice (cauliflower rice instead), feta, oil, and dressing/vinaigrette on salad
- Kabob Family Dinner
  without: sauce, feta, oil, and dressing/vinaigrette on salad
- Mediterranean Chicken Family Dinner
  without: caramelized onions (grilled onions instead), feta, oil, and dressing/vinaigrette on salad

Sides & Snack Boxes

- Seasonal Fresh Fruit
  without: feta, tzatziki, Israeli skhug, oil, and dressing/vinaigrette
- Side Quinoa Salad
  without: feta and dressing/vinaigrette
- Roasted Vegetables
  without: tzatziki, Moroccan harissa, Mediterranean relish, oil, and dressing/vinaigrette
- Power Grains
  without: white rice (brown rice instead, if available)
- Greek Salad
  without: feta, potato salad, and pita bread

Decentralising God

A Restoration of Belief in the West Through The Blockchain

Caleb J. Rowan

TenBooks Publishing

ISBN: 978-1-923379-11-4

Published by Tenbooks Publishing (*10books@proton.me*)

<u>Disclaimer Notice:</u>

By reading this document, the reader agrees that under no circumstances is the author, or publisher responsible for any losses, direct or indirect, that are incurred as a result of the use of the information contained within this document, including, but not limited to, errors, omissions, or inaccuracies.

First Edition: August, 2025

Contents

Author's Note

This book stands with the Church and with every faith that seeks truth. Its primary purpose is to strengthen Christianity by exploring how the tools of our age—especially decentralised technology—can help renew trust, deepen community, and restore belief where it has faded. Any evaluation of church life is offered in the spirit of building up what is good, so that faith may flourish across every corner of society.

It is unfinished by design—a draft of an idea still taking shape. I chose to share it now, rough edges and loose threads intact, because the conversation matters more than waiting for perfection. This is your chance to shape whether it becomes something lasting or just kindling. Thank you for stepping in while it still has dirt under its nails.

—CJ Rowan

Preface

Closer to Church, Further from Christ

We were seated around a long table in a private dining room in the West Indies—C-suite leaders, consultants, and senior advisors. Somewhat unexpectedly, I was asked to say grace before the meal.

I fumbled my way through the only prayer I could remember from childhood:

"For what we are about to receive, may the Lord make us truly thankful. Amen."

It immediately felt awkward. Too short. Sunday-school simple. I mumbled an apology, admitting I wasn't a regular churchgoer and didn't really know what I was doing.

The CEO, a man known for his composure and influence, looked at me without irony and said in a gravelly tone:

"Closer to church, further from Christ."

The table fell silent. A few chuckled nervously, unsure if it was a critique or a blessing.

But the words cut clean through the room—and through something in me.

As a committed Christian, he wasn't mocking faith, but he was clearly mourning something. Mourning the distance between form and essence. Between the appearance of belief and the reality of it. A poetic comparison of systems built around God—with the presence of God Himself.

It named a truth many of us feel but rarely say aloud: that religion, in its institutional form, often builds walls where it once built bridges—places where we can gather in the name of Christ yet walk away untouched by his truth.

This book grapples with that tension and its implications for the future of the West.

It's about our search for something greater than the shell of religion.

Greater than algorithms and performance virtue.

It's about the restoration of something sacred—certainly not new in essence, but radically new in structure.

In a time when institutions are eroding and emerging technologies are reshaping our social fabric, we face an urgent question:

Can faith survive in the West without the control of institutions? Can belief be rebuilt without ownership?

If you're open enough to imagine that the answer to the West's deepest crisis might not come from within the academy, the state, or the market—but from something older, stranger, and still unfolding—then these pages are worth your attention. That maybe, one day, it will also bring a great many in the West back to a deep and fulfilling sense of faith—closer to what's real.

The Whitepaper

When Satoshi Nakamoto published the Bitcoin whitepaper on October 31, 2008, to an obscure cryptography mailing list, it barely caused a ripple. Its core ideas—peer-to-peer currency, proof-of-work, decentralised trust—were understood by only a small circle of cryptographers, cypherpunks, and libertarian technologists. Hal Finney was one of the first to see its potential, mining the first Bitcoin block and receiving the first-ever transaction from Satoshi. Others like Wei Dai (b-money) and Nick Szabo (bit gold) engaged seriously, but most reactions were skeptical, citing issues with scalability, energy use, or the

unresolved double-spend problem. Mainstream economists and tech leaders dismissed it as unrealistic or irrelevant.

But it was enough.

This book may land the same way. A proposal from a pseudonymous author. Faux visionary perhaps, implausible to most. But if even a handful of thinkers—ethicists, theologians, builders—recognise the spark, then the central idea in this book doesn't need to convince the world to begin.

It only needs a few who are willing to fork belief from collapse—and build.

Faith Without a Gatekeeper

We live in an era in the West where belief itself feels broken.

Not just believing in God, but in anything greater than the self.

Institutions are failing us. Our leaders disappoint, all while algorithms distract.

Trust—the binding force of any meaningful culture—is bleeding out, one scandal, one breach, one algorithmic lie at a time.

Does this matter?

Well, yes, it matters very much.

At stake is more than our belief in Christianity. It's the survival of every Western civilisation built upon its foundations.

Institutions and cultural voices with other agendas worked to make what once held people together seem foolish, oppressive, or outdated, replacing it with ideas that promised limitless freedom but left many people feeling lost, with nowhere to go.

For centuries, religion offered order and orientation. Whether or not you were a believer, it anchored societies in shared rituals, moral codes, and transcendent truths.

But those anchors have slipped. Many churches once filled with throngs of worshipers now echo with absence. Increasingly, those architectural masterpieces are being converted into social centres, pri-

vate homes, or falling into disrepair. According to the Pew Research Center, belief in God and regular religious attendance have been in steep decline for decades, especially among younger generations (Pew Research Center, 2018).

We were told that secularism would liberate us. That science, technology, and individual freedom would replace outdated myths. And yet, here we are — more anxious, divided and addicted to outrage and peer approval than ever before.

Many of us no longer know what we stand for — only what we stand against. Into that vacuum rushed new creeds[1].

— Self-branding became a moral compass.

— Fitness routines became spiritual disciplines.

— Political tribes became churches.

— Tech CEOs became prophets.

And yet, deep down, we suspect the truth: *these are weak gods*. They don't satisfy the human need to feel rooted in something enduring, meaningful and shared.

The problem isn't just that many in our societies have lost God. It's that they've lost trust in the institutions that claimed to represent Him. Religious corruption. Abuse scandals. Financial improprieties. Hypocrisy. The rot is well documented. What remains are millions upon millions of spiritual orphans: people who hunger for meaning but refuse to kneel to what they see as broken systems.

So what now? Do we retreat into private belief? Compile personal religions? Wait for something better?

Or — and this is this book's invitation—is it time to reimagine not just what we believe in but also how we might *wrap belief itself in a transparent, tamper-resistant layer that allows trust to scale without control?*

In recent years, blockchain technology has offered new metaphors for trust: distributed, transparent, self-correcting systems, immutable

1. In conventional use, a **creed** is a formal, fixed statement of religious belief or doctrine, often recited collectively and used to define membership or orthodoxy within a faith tradition—like the Nicene Creed in Christianity.

ledgers where truth can't be altered by power or personality, systems where no single entity controls the narrative.

These ideas may sound technical — even cold and unfeeling — but at their heart is something deeply human: *the desire to believe in something incorruptible.*

What if we took the best of a faith like Christianity — its moral compass, a sense of humility before mystery, the call to live for something greater — and rebuilt it on new foundations? What if we could create sacred systems that didn't rely on charismatic leaders or fallible hierarchies, but on shared values encoded into protocols?

What if we could decentralise God?

— not literally; that would be ridiculous, but what if we could decentralise the architecture and systems set up to connect with Him, and worship Him?

This book is not a call to discard tradition. *It is, in fact, an effort to preserve it*—by reimagining how it can endure more broadly. Nor is it a fantasy of techno-utopia. It is a humble and incomplete proposal to imagine what it is that might bring many lapsed believers and non-believers back to faith. To trace the outlines of a faith that cannot be owned, controlled, or corrupted. A faith not bound to any one church, platform, or nation. That evolves without losing its essence.

If that sounds impossible, consider this: *The old maps are already burning.* And those who will thrive in the coming age are not those who cling to the ruins, but those who dare to draw new ones.

But 'belief' is not just personal. It is civilisational. Faith once seeded the very structures we now mourn — schools, hospitals, human rights, even the technologies through which you read these words. Christianity, not consumerism, first declared the dignity of the poor, the sacredness of the stranger, and the moral arc that made abolition thinkable and compassion scalable.

So the question now is not just "Can belief be reborn?" It's: *Can belief be rebooted fast enough to matter?*

Can the protocol become the seed of a new renaissance — before civilisational decline becomes collapse?

Before anyone had heard of Bitcoin, or a blockchain—before the headlines, or the hype—there was just a document. Nine pages of careful thought. A small piece of open-source code. And one silent block, stamped with a line from the news.

What follows here is both a meager blueprint and humble prayer: that the same sacred spark that once lifted humanity from barbarism might ignite again—this time, forked not from empires or priesthoods but from conscience, code, and covenant.

This book begins from the conviction that Christianity's gifts to the West—a deep moral framework, a sense of purpose, and a call to live beyond the self—are worth preserving, rebuilding, and restoring. A decentralised alternative is not a replacement for Christianity but a complement to it, open to participants in any faith tradition who seek truth, trust, and transcendence.

"Geometry is one and eternal, shining in the mind of God. That share in it accorded to men is one of the reasons man is the image of God."[1]

—Johannes Kepler, Dissertatio cum Nuncio Sidereo (1610)

1. Kepler saw geometry as an eternal truth belonging to God alone, yet shared with humanity — unchanging, universal, and beyond the ownership of any one person or power. In the same way, the truth of God is entrusted to all His people to guard, to live by, and to pass on without distortion or doubt.

Introduction

Christian belief in the West hasn't vanished, but it has been pushed to the margins. Many of the institutions that once sustained it have grown hollow—politicised, performative, or compromised—while the West's cultural leaders championed science and reason as if these alone could explain everything. In the process, something greater has been lost: the collapse of transcendence—and with it, the vision to sacrifice the present for the sake of the future, to preserve heritage, to anchor values that could outlast us and serve generations yet to come.

Traditional Faith

For some, the church became too political, performative, or compromised to trust. For others, religion was never an option to begin with—just a dusty leftover from a more gullible age. There's a quiet hunger for meaning, permanence, something that reaches higher than the next outrage or trend. So what might be the way in for unready to join a congregation, but still feel the pull of *something more.*

This book isn't about returning to church, though that would certainly be welcome.

Nor is it about replacing traditional forms of faith—quite the contrary.

Instead it offers a complementary path alongside the Church — a spiritual pressure valve, with moral architecture for those who feel the pull of something more but can't yet walk back into a pew. Something

that will ask whether anything in you still believes there's more to life than metrics, politics, and scrolling.

The truth is, not everyone renounced belief—but many rejected the institutions that claimed to own it. They watched leaders flip their values to stay relevant, while ordinary people were left to either go along or walk away.

Decentralised Faith

Decentralised Faith doesn't pretend to fix all of that. What it does is offer an alternative architecture. One without a central authority that can amend the rules overnight. Instead, it offers something simpler, but more durable: a record of conviction, a space for honest disagreement, a way to participate without surrendering your conscience. Wherever traditional faith has been compromised by power, Decentralised Faith makes power optional—and for the untethered multitudes, that may be the beginning of trust again.

Decentralised Faith isn't a thought experiment. It's technically possible now. At its core is a decentralised protocol—an open-source system of spiritual participation built on blockchain. Trustless, tamper-resistant ledgers record belief, memory, and commitment without hierarchy or middlemen. Smart contracts replace opaque authority with transparent, programmable agreements. Actions are encoded on-chain, whether forming a prayer DAO, witnessing a covenant, or proposing a ritual.

A Genesis Document acts as the foundation—a forkable, open-source spiritual README that defines purpose, principles, and processes. It's stored publicly. Anyone can read it, update it, or fork it. In addition to founding principles, it might contain content from the King James Bible, a distillation of several Biblical texts, or a collection of deeply resonant spiritual teachings.

Nodes are local expressions of faith: communities that gather physically or digitally to pray, reflect, serve, or govern. Some will look like

monasteries, some like message boards, and some might blend both. But each carries forward its part of the chain.

It isn't about charisma or rank. It's earned through visible presence. You build trust by showing up and being counted, pseudonymously or not.

Divergence doesn't erase memory—it preserves it. Communities can part ways when values shift or consensus breaks without destroying their common record that once bound them together.

The Illusion of Immunity

Some point to Islam as a counter-example to Christianity—a religious tradition that seems to resist the demographic collapse of the secular West. And for now, this appears true. Many Muslim-majority countries maintain higher birth rates, tighter communities, and more visible religious identity.

But the trendlines tell a deeper story.

Wherever modernity penetrates—through digital saturation, economic individualism, and consumer-driven culture—birth rates decline, even in strongly religious contexts. We see it now in Iran, Turkey, and increasingly among second- and third-generation Muslim immigrants in the West. The pattern repeats:

— Higher education delays family formation
— Urbanisation weakens clan and community ties
— Affluence trades children for comfort
— Faith becomes symbolic, then optional

Islam may not be the exception. It may simply be the last one standing before modernity finishes its sweep.

The question, then, is not which religion can resist decline. The question is what kind of belief can resist it?

The evidence is overwhelming: Only *embodied faith*—that is lived and practiced daily—has the power to counter the pull of secular drift.

Only a faith that reorders life, rather than decorates it, can resist the logic of materialism, isolation, and decline.

And this applies as much to Christianity as it does to Islam, Judaism, or any enduring tradition. Culture cannot substitute for conviction. Identity cannot stand in for discipline.

When faith is lived, it forms lives that form futures. Without that, even the strongest religious legacy can be hollowed out in a generation or two.

The Return of the Question

For much of the 20th and early 21st century, faith was not just doubted, its value and purpose were increasingly questioned. At elite universities, in pop science books, and across the West's cultural institutions, a new consensus emerged: that the universe was random, life was accidental, and consciousness was just chemistry. Religion, in that view, wasn't just outdated — it was obsolete.

This loss of trust in the Church made the retreat easier. But something else drove it too: the belief that science had closed the old questions.

And yet, with increasing frequency, those questions have returned.

Physicists now speak openly of fine-tuning — a universe so precisely calibrated that even the smallest change would make life impossible. Biologists admit the origins of life remain unsolved — not just improbable, but *unexplainable* by unguided evolution alone. The mystery of consciousness — of *why* there is an inner life at all — remains untouched.

These aren't the arguments of fundamentalists. They come from leading voices within science itself. They do not prove God. But they make it intellectually honest to wonder again.

As the age of certainty recedes, we face an older truth: belief was never eclipsed by knowledge—it was displaced by a culture that privileged literalism over meaning, and calculations over myth. But the human psyche was never wired to live by data alone. Faith speaks the language

of the right hemisphere—symbol, story, and sacrifice—where deep truths lodge deeply, not in logic, but in the will and the soul.

Restoring Belief in the West

This book isn't trying to imagine a new religion. Traditional Christianity still anchors millions—and if anything, Decentralised Faith would strengthen, not replace that. The aim here is simpler and older: to recover something that existed long before churches and doctrines: the instinct to seek meaning, to remember what matters, and to live in a way that honours what's been handed down. Decentralised Faith gives that instinct a home again—in shared memory and everyday commitment.

The West's story is inseparable from the biblical imagination. King Alfred of England drew directly on Hebrew law from the Old Testament in shaping English common law. He saw in those early books not only divine instruction, but the story of a people—family becoming tribe, tribe becoming nation—bound together by covenant. Law was not simply to establish order. It was moral glue.

That vision shaped the very idea of the nation-state. Centuries later, the U.S. Constitution would open with "We the People," echoing the Old Testament's emphasis on forming a unified people rather than a loose collection of individuals.

Enlightenment thinkers such as John Locke reframed this foundation. By placing religion in the realm of individual conscience and grounding the state in neutrality and equality before the law, Locke secured liberty of conscience. But the shift carried a cost. Once neutrality replaced covenant as the state's bedrock, the unity of the West rested on procedure rather than shared moral inheritance.

The decline of Christianity's public influence became an inevitability.

Any reversal requires a return to something older: the instinct to seek, to remember, to live in ways that honour what was handed down. That instinct deserves a structure built for this era.

Blockchain?

If you've never heard of blockchain applied to faith, you're not alone, but the idea isn't without precedent. Thinkers and labs like Sacred Design Lab are already experimenting with rituals for the spiritually unaffiliated—proof that the hunger remains, even if the forms shift. Projects like Raiinmaker have gone a step further, testing AI-driven spiritual advisors. But what's missing in those efforts isn't intelligence—it's reverence. They reveal more about our ache for connection than they do about architecture that can truly hold belief. What's needed isn't simulated sanctity, but systems of trust built to carry spiritual weight.

Scholar Jonny Stryder's *Blockchain Faith* imagined how ledgers and public consensus could serve justice and distributed accountability. But sacredness—the rituals, the memory, the sense of presence—is largely absent from that vision. If Stryder sketches the civic square, this book steps into the chapel beside it.

And for those who've read Charles Eisenstein's *Sacred Economics*, this is not a departure, but an extension. Eisenstein reminded a generation that markets must serve meaning, not the other way around. He re-sacralised value through the language of gift. But the digital age asks new questions: How do we remember covenant? How do we protect the sacred from manipulation, not just commodification? *Decentralising God* builds on that momentum, offering permanence where institutions fray, and protocols where hierarchies once stood.

This is not the only attempt to restore trust in the spiritual domain, but it may be one of the few that begins with architecture, not authority, and with consent, not pronouncement. If nothing else, let this book be proof that the ache for something greater hasn't gone quiet. It's still here—dispersed, maybe, but no less real. And perhaps that's the point: faith doesn't need to be loud to last. It needs to be lived.

But if you've ever felt the tug that there must be more than this—more than noise, more than self, more than the here and

now—then maybe this is your place to start. Toward something "greater than" ourselves. Something transcendent.

Faith doesn't need to be loud to last. It just needs to be embodied.

A Natural Next Step in Christian Renewal: Decentralised Faith

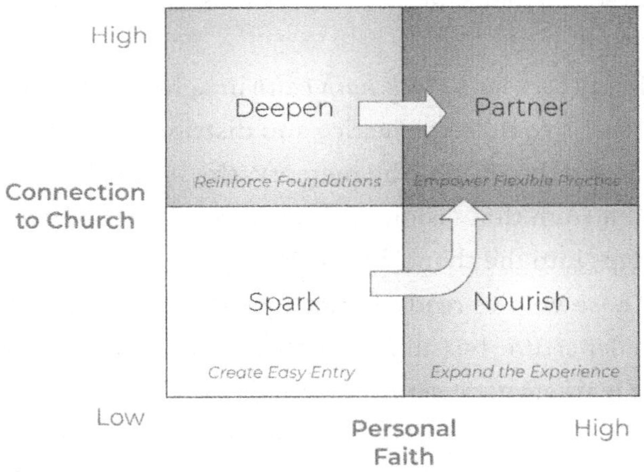

Goal: *Restore and Reinforce Lived Christian Faith in the West*

Aim: *Revive and reinforce lived Christian faith so it once again anchors Western culture.*

Role of Decentralised Faith: High trust, memory, coordination, and consent-based practice.

SIDE BAR: Decline—What the Data Shows[1]

Across disciplines, the pattern is consistent:
– *Practicing* religious groups sustain higher fertility & social cohesion
– *Nominal* or inherited faith collapses under modern individualism
– Civilisations that forget this pattern tend to decline demographically and culturally

These are not marginal findings. They are well-established across history and culture. The question is no longer whether faith matters. The question is whether it's still lived.

1. **Sources:**
– Pew Research (2015–2021)
– Lyman Stone, Institute for Family Studies
– Eric Kaufmann, *Shall the Religious Inherit the Earth?*
– Philip Jenkins, *The Next Christendom*
– Rodney Stark, *The Rise of Christianity*

Build Systems They Cannot Erase

What follows is a short but important aside. While this book is primarily about spiritual decentralisation, the same principles can safeguard something just as vital to a civilisation's health: its cultural memory.

> *What survives is what the powerful permit—unless we build systems they cannot erase.*

Preserving Cultural Memory Without Permission

In the United Kingdom at the date of publishing, debates around the Online Safety Bill have raised concerns about the quiet erasure of certain historical episodes from public curricula or digital archives. Reports suggest that topics like the Crusades are being de-emphasised—or avoided entirely—on the grounds that they might offend particular groups. Whether or not the intent is malicious, the result is the same: cultural memory becomes selectively edited, often by those with little accountability.

Another powerful application of the decentralised faith model that follows lies in its design. The same principles—open protocols, distributed stewardship, and cryptographic integrity—could preserve far more than sacred records, safeguarding Western cultural works, contested histories, and primary sources that might otherwise be altered, hidden, or erased.

A blockchain ledger can store metadata and verification proofs for any document, image, or dataset, ensuring authenticity over decades or centuries. GitHub-style repositories allow collaborative maintenance of these works, with every change visible and reversible—no hidden edits, no silent deletions. Decentralised file systems like IPFS (InterPlanetary File System) or Arweave store the actual content across thousands of independent nodes, making it almost impossible for any single authority to remove it. Even if a government, corporation, or platform de-indexes or bans the material, the network still carries it.

In such a system, students could access a verifiable copy of a historical source—be it a medieval charter, a banned novel, or an archive of political speeches—knowing that it has not been altered. Teachers, researchers, and ordinary citizens could fork repositories, add context, annotate, and share without fear of losing the original record. Just as the printing press—championed by many within the Church—broke the monopoly on written scripture, these decentralised tools break the monopoly on cultural memory.

Preserving history in this way isn't about resisting sensitivity or ignoring the harm in certain narratives. It's about refusing to let any one generation, ideology, or committee decide which parts of our shared story get to survive. In a world where "offensive" can mean "unwelcome to power," distributed preservation may be the only way to ensure that the past remains whole enough for the future to judge.

A Note on Names & Terms

"The naming of things is a difficult matter."

T.S. Eliot

No name is final. In true decentralised fashion, it'll be forked, evolved, and collectively refined.

Language is always late to the party. When something new is stirring, we reach for old words to make sense of it. But the containers we borrow—faith, church, belief, community—come with layers of architecture and history. Terms that once felt raw and relational now carry the weight of centuries.

This book doesn't try to solve that. It explores the idea of a decentralised spiritual movement—faith without institutional gatekeepers, but what do we call it?

"D-Faith" is the placeholder used throughout this book. It's clunky, but it doesn't need to be elegant. It just needs to serve a role while something more universally resonant emerges. Some will read "D" as decentralised, others as distributed, or even disintermediated. That ambiguity is intentional.

Other names hover at the edges:

— *Bit-Faith*

— *Chainfaith*

— *Soulchain*

— *Sacred Protocol*

—*Distributed Church*

—*Proof-of-Spirit*

Each one captures a facet. None is complete.

Even in Scripture, names changed with purpose—Abram became Abraham, Jacob became Israel[1], Saul came to be known as Paul. And before they were called Christians, the first believers were simply known as *the Way*.

In a decentralised world, language can fork too.

Consider this a first attempt—unfinished, Version 1.0.

Common Christian Terms, Reimagined for D-Faith

Communion: Traditionally, a ritual of bread and wine shared in sacred presence. In D-Faith, it's presence too—offered by co-signing, witnessing, or contributing to the ledger. Trust, without mediation.

Covenant: Once a solemn pact, made sacred by God or scripture. Now, a voluntary commitment—recorded openly, bound by integrity, held together by mutual memory.

Creed: Fixed words once spoken to prove belief. Here, a creed is chosen. Signed. Visible. Not enforced—but trusted.

Liturgy: Ritual once scheduled and led by clergy. Now, code can carry it. Protocols of prayer, renewal, and repair—coordinated by community.

Revelation: Once delivered, declared, and closed. Now open. Ongoing. Truth shared and refined in public view.

Sacred: Traditionally, what was declared holy. Now, what we refuse to discard. What we handle with care because it matters.

1. i.e. **Jacob** ▯ **Israel** – In Genesis 32:28, Jacob wrestles with a divine being and is renamed Israel ("he struggles with God)

Transcendence: The divine beyond. Now also the long view: planting for those we'll never meet. Writing truths meant to last.

Witness: To see and testify to what's holy. Still true. But now, shared. To witness is to honour and confirm—together.

PART I: COLLAPSE & CRITIQUE

The Modern West

"Do you not know that you *are God's temple and that God's Spirit dwells in* you?"

— 1 Corinthians 3:16

Chapter 1

The Age of Hollow Metrics

Drowning in data. Starving for meaning.

Core Problem or Tension: We are surrounded by metrics, measurements, and KPIs—but starving for meaning. The modern world has mistaken quantity for quality, and visibility for value.

What This Chapter Offers: This chapter critiques the dominance of reductive metrics in culture, economics, and identity. It invites readers to recognize the limitations of data-driven thinking and consider how spiritual and moral truths resist quantification.

Why It Matters Now: In an age of dashboards and surveillance, we're losing touch with what actually matters. This chapter lays the groundwork for reclaiming meaning that isn't measurable but is essential.

> *"The madman is not the man who has lost his reason. The madman is the man who has lost everything except his reason."*
>
> G.K. Chesterton

At some point in the last few decades, we fell in love with what we can measure.

Once, we prayed for guidance. Today, we bow our heads to the modest glow of a screen, waiting for an answer shaped by invisible logic. It feels neutral—even divine—but these responses reflect learned behaviour, not wisdom. They mirror us, but they do not raise us.

Our ancestors lit candles. We refresh tabs.

We no longer ask, *"What is good?"* but *"What performs?"* The algorithm is not evil, but it is indifferent—and its reach is now more intimate than any pastoral conversation or confession.

What began as a tool became a worldview. If it could be counted, it counted. Productivity, net worth, test scores, calories, followers, GDP—our new commandments. And yet the truth slips quietly through: the numbers are empty.

The Illusion of Progress

Our children ace exams yet cannot sleep. We climb career ladders and wonder why the summit feels hollow. The more we chase metrics, the more we lose sight of what we were aiming for in the first place.

Ivan Illich warned that tools begin to control us when they stop serving purpose. We are there now.

A teacher once told me, "I used to shape humans. Now I prep them for multiple-choice questions." The metrics insist students are improving, but their own voices tell another story—anxiety, burnout, and disengagement.

Social media rewards outrage, not truth. We learn to look real but forget how to feel real. In healthcare, patients notice when the doctor never quite meets their eyes. They may leave with a prescription, but not always a sense that they were seen.

Measurement helps, but it was never meant to lead. And when it leads, it often warps. We end up counting what's easy, not what's vital.

What Cannot Be Counted

Even grief gets flattened into a signal—an icon tapped, a string of reactions. But does the one in mourning feel less alone?

We arrange our lives to suit what machines can register, and in doing so, we sideline what only the human spirit can hold. This is more than spiritual drift; it is the slow redrawing of our inner compass.

Wisdom is not a poll result.

Virtue does not parade itself.

What is sacred resists the scan.

Love, loyalty, awe, sacrifice—these are the soil beneath our feet. Numbers may trace the outline of a life, but they cannot approach its substance.

When everything must be measured, we begin to value only the measurements. And that, as Chesterton saw, is the first step into madness.

Chapter 2

The Age of Me

Core Problem or Tension: We've made the self the ultimate guide for meaning and purpose, but it wasn't built for that burden—leaving many of us anxious, alone, and adrift.

What This Chapter Offers: A critique of hyper-individualism and therapeutic culture. It explores how the elevation of the self—while empowering in some ways—has undermined our capacity for belonging, sacrifice, and transcendence.

Why It Matters Now: Self-obsession is marketed as self-care, and identity is treated as destiny. This chapter calls for a rediscovery of meaning beyond the mirror—for communities, for traditions, for something greater.

"We are now living in a spiritual supernova, a kind of galloping pluralism on every level."

— Charles Taylor, A Secular Age (2007)

We live in an age that treats the self as sacred. What began as a rightful correction—affirming dignity, voice, and autonomy—has hardened into something heavier. Ads sell us back to ourselves. Algorithms finish our thoughts. Institutions bow to choice instead of standing on principle.

There's justice in this shift. For centuries, hierarchy silenced individuals. At times, religion's structures obscured the very soul they were meant to nurture. The modern embrace of self-worth was a reckoning. But somewhere, the self became not just important but untouchable.

Eric Hoffer warned that, "*Every great cause begins as a movement, becomes a business, and eventually degenerates into a racket.*". Expressive individualism is no exception. We embraced 'freedom' and increasingly found ourselves alone.

The U.S. Surgeon General, Dr. Vivek Murthy, has called loneliness a public health crisis. Chronic isolation raises the risk of early death, yet more people than ever feel unseen. Social media broadcasts us but rarely binds us. Sherry Turkle observed that we now live with "the illusion of companionship without the demands of friendship."

Even our morality feels digitised. Autocomplete doesn't just finish sentences—it steers convictions. Spotify reads your mood. Google anticipates your fears. We are told to "follow our truth," but not where it leads.

This is the core of expressive individualism, a term popularised by Robert Bellah: moral authority comes from within. The highest good is to be "true to yourself." But when the self becomes source, solution, and sacred object, it buckles under the weight.

Commitment feels like captivity, sacrifice looks like betrayal. Marriage, parenting, friendship, and even faith are reframed as lifestyle options, similarly curated like playlists. We teach people to 'find' themselves but not to *lose* themselves in something greater.

The data is catching up to the experience. Teenage sadness and anxiety are at historic highs. We gave them endless tools for expression. We did not provide them with anything to belong to.

The self matters. But it is not enough.

Every enduring tradition has known this. In Buddhism, the self is an illusion. In Christianity, it is surrendered. In Judaism, it is fulfilled in covenant. In Islam, it is quieted before God.

Faith doesn't erase the self—it gives it proportion.

Modern spirituality, by contrast, seeks transcendence without demand, connection without cost, and meaning without responsibility. We've mistaken spiritual autonomy for maturity.

So, where do we go from here?

First, honesty.

The self is authentic, but not final—it's a good beginning, but never a god.

Next, humility.

The self cannot bear the burden of ultimate meaning.

There is structure. Not a reimagining of hierarchical control, but a renewed architecture—one that protects dignity while restoring connection, in harmony with the life of the Church. This is where decentralised faith begins to speak.

D-Faith is not a rejection of the self—it is a re-anchoring. You are a node, not the whole network. Vital, but not sovereign.

The sacred isn't found in self-expression alone. It lives in covenant, in action and commitment—many safeguarded and deepened by the Church—that outlast ego.

The Age of Me gave us exposure without intimacy. We are saturated with self, yet starved for belonging.

The self doesn't need tearing down—only lifting: Toward others, and toward the transcendent.

Finally, the architecture of D-Faith reframes the conditions of belief—what Charles Taylor calls the space in which faith is even possible—so that existing traditions, including the Church, can thrive alongside new expressions. This design protects dignity while restoring connection, shifting the self from being the whole horizon to being part of a shared world. This is where decentralised faith begins to speak.

Chapter 3

The State, the Market, and the Void

Core Problem or Tension: As trust in spiritual traditions waned, modern societies outsourced meaning-making to the State and the Market. But these institutions were never designed to bear that spiritual load.

What This Chapter Offers: A historical and cultural examination of how bureaucratic governance and consumer capitalism stepped into the vacuum once filled by faith—and why they fall short. It highlights the spiritual emptiness of systems focused on control and consumption.

Why It Matters Now: Neither politics nor commerce can offer transcendence. Yet both compete for our loyalty, shaping our desires and beliefs. Reclaiming a moral and sacred framework beyond these forces is critical to human flourishing.

> *"We had fed the heart on fantasies, The heart's grown brutal from the fare."*
> — W.B. Yeats, Meditations in Time of Civil War (1922)

Once, people believed kings ruled by divine right—that justice came from above and order reflected something sacred, not merely social.

Even when abused, those beliefs held society together—not because they were flawless, but because they aimed beyond themselves.

The modern West let go of that anchor.

To end religious conflict, we turned to the state—neutral, procedural, meant to referee rather than rule. Thinkers like Hobbes and Locke imagined law replacing faith as our shared ground. For a while, it worked. Liberal democracy became the new sacred.

But over time, the state was asked to do more—not just govern but validate, not just protect rights but provide purpose. We expected it to fix everything, then grew bitter when it couldn't. Trust cracked. Polarisation set in.

Into that vacuum stepped the market.

Where the state promised fairness, the market promised choice. It delivered endless convenience and innovation—and relative global prosperity. Yet, markets reward engagement, not wisdom. What sells best often distracts or divides.

Consumerism became a kind of civil religion—brands as identity, shopping as ritual, endless desires to be satisfied.

Still, the deeper questions remain:

Why are we here?

What does a good life require?

To whom—or what—do we belong?

That's the void.

And into it flood anxiety, addiction, and ideology. Religion hasn't vanished, but in some contexts it has been repurposed—drawn into cultural combat rather than nurtured for spiritual depth. Belief turns brittle. Sacred texts become weapons.

Sociologists Christian Smith and Melinda Denton call the default faith of many young people *Moralistic Therapeutic Deism*: a vague belief in a distant God who mainly wants us to be nice. No challenge. No covenant. No transformation.

We drift. Some cling harder to tradition, while others abandon it. Many convert politics or self-help into religion. However, none of these fill the space meaning once held, because none are deeply relational.

We've built systems without soul: governance without grace, freedom without formation, choice without cohesion.

And the house shakes.

Despite endless stimulation and novelty, people are still searching for something steady, with depth. You see it in the return to ritual, the draw toward Orthodoxy, and the hunger for philosophies like Stoicism. Beneath the noise, people want *structure that matters*—something worthy of reverence, even when it comes at a cost.

But the state can't offer it. The market won't. They were never designed to.

When a society loses the sacred, it doesn't become wise—it becomes angry. Rage replaces awe. We grasp at tribe when tradition fails, but tribalism without shared moral ground eventually devolves into suspicion and contempt.

That's the real crisis: a community without commitment breed identity without intimacy and belonging based on opposition (by *who or what you stand against)*.

What's needed is not more spectacle, but re-sacralisation.

Frameworks that voluntarily bind—by meaning. Faith that decentralises power, distributes memory, and rebuilds trust through integrity.

This is where decentralised faith begins to matter. Its aim is not to replace the Church or any living tradition, but to strengthen and preserve the sacred where it has been thinned, offering tools that serve renewal.

If blockchain can secure value, why not sacred memory?

If it can distribute consensus, why not covenant?

If it can resist corruption, why not spiritual control?

Faith need not be housed only in systems that are vulnerable to breaking.

It can be peer-to-peer. Witnessed. Durable. Alive.

The state was never meant to be our priest, and it cannot carry that role.

The market was never meant to be our god, and it cannot bear that weight.

And the void will not wait.

From more than a century ago, Yeats words echo even more powerfully today:

> *"Things fall apart; the center cannot hold;*
> *Mere anarchy is loosed upon the world,*
> *The blood□dimmed tide is loosed, and everywhere*
> *The ceremony of innocence is drowned;*
> *The best lack all conviction, while the worst*
> *Are full of passionate intensity."*

Chapter 4

The Decline of Shared Myth in the West

When Stories No Longer Bind Us

Core Problem or Tension: A culture without myth is a culture without meaning. In rejecting shared stories, we've lost the frameworks that once guided identity, sacrifice, and hope.

What This Chapter Offers: An examination of how myths functioned as moral architecture and why their collapse has left us fragmented. It invites re-engagement with symbolic language and story.

Why It Matters Now: Without shared myths, we struggle to connect generations, build communities, or sacrifice for the common good. This chapter sets the stage for reimagining spiritual story.

> *"Where myth disappears, meaning collapses—and barbarism soon follows."*
>
> — George Steiner, Real Presences (1989)

There was a time when the stories people shared weren't just for entertainment. They helped hold communities together and gave shape to memory, grief and duty. They reminded each generation why life mattered—and how to live it well.

These weren't just tales passed down at bedtime. They ran deeper. In Aboriginal Australia, the Dreaming spoke of ancestors and land in one breath. In the Gita, a warrior's hesitation carried the weight of moral clarity. Genesis didn't just start a religion—it framed how millions understood time, truth, and responsibility.

These stories didn't ask to be proven, only to be remembered.

Now those stories have frayed. And in their absence, we feel the drift.

Today, "myth" often means a falsehood. But in anthropology, a myth is a truth carried in narrative form—a moral map, a way to hold what facts alone cannot. Joseph Campbell called myths "public dreams," the narratives that help us metabolise death, longing, love, and loss. They teach morality to the young without a sermon. They explain purpose without a diagram. Myths give us a place in the world—not just geographically, but spiritually.

For centuries, the West lived in the afterglow of a Judeo-Christian mythos. Even those outside the Church carried its moral grammar: the inherent value of the individual, the redemptive arc of history, the binding power of covenant, the centrality of truth—gifts the Church has carried and preserved through the centuries. But that shared grammar is dissolving. Religious literacy declines. Public rites grow secular. Generational memory scatters.

What replaces it? A noise of competing truths—personal brands, niche ideologies, micro-narratives.

Carl Jung warned: *The man who thinks he can live without myth is already ensnared by one—his own.*

Everyone has a story now, but we lack a shared story. Without it, even good people lose the plot because there is no common plot to follow. So we craft meaning from hashtags, protests, subscriptions, and unsubscribes. These new myths can rally us, but rarely root us. They tell us who to oppose, not who to become.

The dominant myth of the modern West has been progress. For a time, it delivered science, literacy, rights, and abundance. But it carried unspoken assumptions—that growth is endless, that "freedom", or at

least the perception of being free, is enough, and that technology can replace community. Freedom without purpose becomes drift. Individualism without belonging becomes fracture.

We don't need nostalgia. We need a story that feels both ancient and unfinished—one that honours the faith traditions that shaped us while opening space for renewal.

What if faith could be decentralised—to serve and strengthen?

What if wisdom could be shared?

What if covenant could be encoded—not to control, but to secure commitment?

Blockchain is more than code. It is memory that resists corruption, in a structure that persists.

If Steiner is correct, then the erosion of our shared myths is not just a cultural loss—it is an open invitation to collapse.

Myths don't die—they adapt. And the right story, told well and lived honestly, could yet remind us who we are.

Chapter 5

What Is D-Faith?

The sacred, without the gatekeepers.

Core Problem or Tension: People are seeking spiritual belonging, but many no longer trust the traditional gatekeepers. Institutional religion can feel distant, political, or commodified.

What This Chapter Offers: An introduction to D-Faith—the idea that sacred meaning, memory, and moral accountability can be distributed without being diluted. It's not anti-religion; it's post-gatekeeping.

Why It Matters Now: Technology has created new ways to organise, trust, and remember. This chapter argues that those same tools—blockchain, DAOs, open-source code—can underpin a new kind of spiritual infrastructure.

> *"The aim is not to replace institutions with chaos, but with better protocols."*
>
> — Vitalik Buterin

The question isn't whether people have faith. It's where they place it.

Some trust in God. Others in science, the market, or love. Faith—understood as belief in something beyond immediate proof—isn't rare. It's the bridge we walk when certainty ends. We trust the sun will rise,

the people we love will remain, and the fragile systems we inhabit will hold just long enough for us to act.

But the institutions that once anchored that trust—the church, government, media, even truth itself—are shedding credibility. People rarely abandon belief because they've stopped caring. More often, they leave because the covenant was breached: in some contexts, a church replacing sober conviction with political theatre, a pastor chasing trends, or leaders urging affirmations that seem at odds with historic teaching—moments that, for some, eroded trust. These moments don't just test loyalty; they alter the trust structure.

Permissionless Faith

More people now call themselves "spiritual but not religious." They're not rejecting the sacred; they're stepping away from systems they felt claimed to own it. Scandal, control, and institutional drift weren't side notes—they were the breaking points.

But the search continues. They still pray, even if silently. They still want meaning, connection, and reverence—without the hidden levers.

What if spiritual life could be rebuilt around verifiable trust and shared wisdom, instead of personality or power? That's the heart of D-Faith.

What D-Faith Is (and Isn't)

D-Faith stands for **Decentralised Faith**. It is not a religion in the doctrinal sense; it is an *infrastructure for belief*.

Trust doesn't have to be the byproduct of central control. In distributed systems, trust emerges from consensus—nodes (people, in this case) verifying each other's commitments against a shared ledger.

In blockchain terms:

- **Identity** is anchored in asymmetric cryptography. Each participant holds a *private key*—their ability to sign commitments—and a *public key*—their verifiable identity on the net-

work.

- **Consensus** replaces decrees. Instead of one authority deciding what is "true," multiple participants validate it through protocols such as Proof of Participation or Byzantine Fault Tolerance.

- **Memory** is distributed. Commitments, covenants, and doctrinal forks are stored immutably across the network, resistant to erasure or revisionism.

D-Faith means:

— Participatory meaning-making that can work alongside existing theology, not only top-down forms

— Open-source tradition that honours enduring doctrine while allowing shared stewardship

— Shared rituals that can complement existing rules and traditions

—Trust that lives in transparency

This is not spiritual anarchy. It's distributed reverence—a collective covenant recorded and verified without coercion. And yes, decentralised systems can drift, but the same architecture that enables authentic freedom also provides a forensic memory of divergence.

Why Now?

Spiritual history shifts when trust fractures. The Reformation rose when monopoly failed; the Enlightenment followed when inherited authority cracked.

Today's rupture is digital. The tools that gave us instant communication also centralised narrative control—social algorithms, surveillance models, proprietary platforms. People are tired of communities mediated by black-box systems.

Meanwhile, millions are already experimenting with distributed governance:

- **Decentralised Autonomous Organisations (DAOs)** coordinating global projects without a central board
- **Tokenised trust circles** that reward participation rather than extraction
- **Zero-Knowledge Proofs (ZKPs)** enabling accountability without sacrificing privacy

It's chaotic, but the tools are here.

The Sacred—Shared

For centuries, sacred authority was kept in temples, inscribed in scrolls, and stewarded through hierarchy. That architecture could preserve truth, but at times was also vulnerable to capture.

In D-Faith, a covenant could be a signed transaction: a block in a public ledger, timestamped, verified by the community, and permanently retrievable. Forks—when part of the community diverges—don't erase the past; they copy the entire record so both streams of belief retain the original lineage.

Theologian John D. Caputo once wrote, *"God does not exist. God insists."* In protocol terms, God is not a central server but a persistent process that continues to execute whenever justice and love are instantiated in the network.

What D-Faith Isn't

D-Faith seeks to offer tools that strengthen and preserve the Church and other living traditions, especially in places where trust has been weakened.

This is not a cult.

Or a crypto grift.

Or a vague swirl of slogans.

It's a serious proposal that belief can evolve, trust can be reimagined, and reverence can be shared—without collapsing into chaos.

Signs of Life

It's already emerging:

— Decentralised prayer networks run on distributed ledgers

— Smart-contract covenants triggering action on agreed dates or events

— Myth-making platforms where narrative forks are version-controlled like open-source software

Some will fail. But the hunger is real.

An Open Invitation

D-Faith isn't a finished blueprint. It's a live experiment in protocol design:

—What if Belief didn't require obedience?

—What if reverence didn't require hierarchy?

—What if belonging could be verified, without being controlled?

It's not certainty. But it's a place to start.

A way to rebuild what still matters—and keep it incorruptible.

Vitalik Buterin reminds us: the aim is not to replace institutions with chaos, but with better protocols.

In faith as in code, the challenge is not merely to remove what is broken, but to build what can endure. D-Faith is merely a thought-bubble, in time the open-source alpha of something larger—an architecture of trust, memory, and reverence that anyone can help improve. Like the best protocols, it will thrive, not because it is perfect, but because it can be forked, refined, and 'lived' into maturity.

The question is not whether belief will adapt. It always has. The question is whether we will have the courage to write the next chapter together, line by line, block by block, in a ledger that tells the truth and makes it worth remembering.

10 Primal Needs Met by D-Faith

At the heart of every spiritual tradition are the same primal questions. D-Faith seeks to meet them in a form fit for this age.

1. **Belonging on Your Terms:** This speaks directly to people burned by coercive community, gatekeeping, or tribal religion. It protects conscience while still inviting commitment, community, and shared purpose. It combines the hunger for spiritual belonging with the right to walk away. **Freedom + depth = high appeal.**

2. **Trust Without Charisma:** Many are exhausted by personality-driven faith, such as celebrity pastors, scandal-ridden leaders, or constant reinvention. This message says *you don't need to follow a guru to belong to something sacred.*

3. **Steadfastness Against Trends:** This hits home for those who feel their churches have compromised to stay relevant. It offers continuity without calcification. A haven for the *traditionally rooted but not reactionary.*

4. **Immutable Memory:** Powerful for those who fear that truth, history, or sacredness is being erased or reinterpreted at will. Appeals to people who want their story to last and their community to remember it honestly.

5. **Forking Without Excommunication:** This needs a little explanation, but once grasped, it's liberating. It reframes divergence as fidelity to conscience, not betrayal. Especially appeal-

ing to those who've had to "quietly leave" communities, or are no longer "all in".

6. **Participation Without Permission:** Subtly robust—especially for women, laypeople, and others who've been told to stay in the pews and let the leaders speak. It opens up the system without diluting its sacredness.

7. **Belief Without Branding:** This is relevant for the spiritually sincere who are weary of churches trying to be social clubs or TED Talk venues. It reassures them that faith can be real without being performative.

8. **Transparency Without Surveillance:** This appeals more to the *technically literate* or institutionally suspicious. It's important, but doesn't hit the heart until trust is already broken.

9. **Freedom Without Chaos:** This sounds abstract until someone worries about fragmentation. It's a good reassurance *after* someone's already interested, but not a front-door message.

10. **Disagreement Without Disintegration:** Important for community builders and theologians—but emotionally less immediate to those just seeking meaning or belonging.

Q: *What kind of Human energy does faith unlock—compared to wealth or fame?*

A: Some systems are powered by money. Some by recognition. But faith—genuine, lived faith—unleashes a different kind of energy altogether.

It's the kind of energy that, in the Church, built cathedrals without deadlines, moved people to carve beauty into ceilings they'd never see, and in the digital age draws coders to anonymous message boards, writing protocols not to receive praise but out of conviction.

We often underestimate what belief can sustain. When someone is moved by meaning, they keep showing up—even when no one's counting. Even when there's no reward but the work itself.

Yes, commercial incentives scale quickly, but they fade when the funding dries up or the spotlight shifts. Faith endures differently. It builds slowly, often invisibly, but what it creates tends to last.

If it's to thrive, D-Faith won't rely on fame or finance. It will depend on an exponentially more potent force—the energy of conviction. The kind that doesn't burn out, because it doesn't begin in ego. It starts in purpose. This is the same enduring current that has sustained the Church for centuries—and which D-Faith seeks to channel into forms that serve renewal today.

For a deeper exploration, read "The Energy of Belief—Conviction over Capital" in the Bonus Materials.

Chapter 6

Closer to Church, Further from Christ

Core Problem or Tension: Institutional religion is more accessible than ever, yet spiritual disconnection persists. Churches remain, but for many, faith feels hollow.

What This Chapter Offers: A nuanced critique of how religious institutions sometimes obscure, rather than illuminate, the sacred. It explores the gap between institutional loyalty and authentic belief.

Why It Matters Now: As scandals, power dynamics, and cultural shifts erode trust in institutions, many walk away from religion altogether. This chapter argues for a faith that can survive without centralisation. Or even complement conventional faith practices, keeping the institutions more honest.

> *"These people honor me with their lips, but their hearts are far from me. They worship me in vain; their teachings are merely human rules."*
>
> Jesus, quoting Isiah (Matthew 15:8–9, NIV)

Something strange is happening across the modern West.

People still say they believe in God—or at least in something greater—but fewer trust Christianity to help them find Him. Churches

empty. Vocations decline. Fewer children inherit the faith of their parents.

And yet, spiritual hunger hasn't vanished. It appears in yoga studios, protest movements, psychedelic retreats, astrology accounts, and self-help podcasts that sound more like sermons than science. We still long for the sacred, but fewer than ever trust the institutions, clergy, or rules that claim to guard it.

For some, religion—once experienced as a source of meaning, morality, and belonging—has felt, at times, like an obstacle to all three. Some even leave church, not because they've lost belief, but because they're trying to preserve it.

The numbers are stark. In 1948, only 2% of Americans told Gallup they had no religious affiliation. Today, it's around 30%, even higher among the young. Christianity fell from 74% in 1991 to 44% in 2021 in Australia. The UK and Canada show similar declines. These aren't small dips; they signal cultural unraveling.

But this isn't just secularisation. It's de-institutionalisation.

Some leave over scandal, others over silence or irrelevance, and many because their doubts met shame instead of curiosity. One woman told me, *"I didn't stop believing in God. I just couldn't recognise what I was being sold in His name."* That line captures our moment: a slow, quiet uncoupling of faith from form.

Faith as an Encounter

For centuries, spiritual life was structured by institutions. Churches didn't just teach belief—they organised it. They set the calendar, held the records, guarded the language of reverence. That world is dissolving.

Now, the tools once kept behind stained glass—scripture, sermons, songs—are everywhere. You don't need a priest or a pew. Access feels open by default. The old gatekeepers are redundant.

But freedom without shared memory is fragile. Belief becomes a mosaic of fragments—quotes, podcasts, memes. It can inspire but of-

ten lacks depth, formation, and the ballast of something larger than personal preference.

Charles Taylor calls this the "immanent frame," a space where belief is contested and optional. James K.A. Smith describes "secular liturgies"—habits like scrolling, shopping, or self-performance—that shape desire while naming nothing sacred. In this way, people are still religious; they've simply traded cathedrals for CrossFit. But CrossFit does not wrestle with eternity.

The phrase "*spiritual but not religious*" carries pride, but beneath it is a plea—for wonder without dogma, connection without control. Diana Butler Bass calls this a move from religion as institution to faith as encounter: less hierarchy, more honesty, closer to the root.

The earliest Christians had no cathedrals or clerical bureaucracy. They gathered in homes, shared meals, and remembered. Their faith was decentralised by necessity. Could it be again—by design?

It Belongs to the Many

The breakdown of trust is not a cue for repair alone; it's an opening for redesign.

The same systems that secure decentralised finance or manage distributed networks can also protect sacred trust, because the underlying challenge is the same: how to coordinate people and preserve memory without a single point of control.

In practice, this means:

- **Distributed record-keeping**: sacred commitments, liturgical changes, and shared decisions logged on a network where no single node can alter the past without consensus.

- **Multi-signature authority**: no one leader holds the "keys" to doctrinal or practical changes; they require collective sign-off, ensuring power remains diffused.

- **Versioned tradition**: when beliefs or practices diverge, each

branch retains the full history—forking preserves continuity rather than erasing it.

These are design patterns for trust. Blockchain, DAOs, and smart contracts are simply the modern tools that make them possible.

Institutions have their place, but they are vulnerable—susceptible to capture, drift, and betrayal. Decentralisation isn't a cure-all, but it resists these specific failures by ensuring no one person or council can rewrite the sacred record for all.

This is more than technical elegance; it reflects a theological claim: The sacred is entrusted to the whole Body—it is stewarded by the many, not owned by the few.

For Those Inside and Out

D-Faith complements tradition—providing tools that can strengthen both the faithful who remain within traditional structures and those searching for a way back.

This is not a rejection of religion. For those nourished by tradition, your place is sacred. But this also offers a way back for the spiritually homeless—those who still long for God but cannot find Him in the old rooms.

Institutions may fade, but the ache for God does not. And that longing deserves a form that cannot betray it—a covenant with both human warmth and cryptographic backbone.

In the gospels, Jesus entrusted His message to friends, not functionaries—scattering it like seed, knowing that truth would take root in many soils. He never wrote a line of scripture Himself, yet His words endured because they were carried, remembered, and retold by the many. A decentralised faith is consistent with that pattern—trusting that it does not weaken when the sacred is shared. It multiplies.

11 Benefits D-Faith Promises:

(Where Traditional Christianity Has Sometimes Struggled)

1. **Unforgettable Memory:** What was once redacted, forgotten, or spun is now preserved—immutable, visible, incorruptible.

2. **Forking Without Shame:** Disagree? Diverge. No excommunication, or erasure—just spiritual integrity on record.

3. **Trust Without Celebrities:** Authority is earned, not assigned. No pulpit power plays. Reputation over time.

4. **Belief Without Branding:** No need to market your convictions. You belong by showing up, not selling out.

5. **Transparency Without Exposure:** Decisions stay visible. Abuses exposed. Privacy stays intact.

6. **Participation Without Gatekeepers:** No title required. Integrity and contribution are paramount.

7. **Conviction Without Drift:** Stay rooted. No central body can force your values to move.

8. **Freedom With Form:** Structure. Covenant. A decentralised structure that still holds shape.

9. **Disagreement Without Collapse:** Conflict remains on record. Seen, held, and endured—without splitting apart.

10. **Community Without Borders:** Join by values, not zip code. Worship across time zones, not institutions.

11. **Consent-Based Belonging:** Free of coercion. Leaving not punished. Free, conscious alignment.

Chapter 7

The Blockchain as Sacred Ledger

Not all holy books are bound in leather. Some are mined, not printed.

Core Problem or Tension: Sacred memory and moral record-keeping are crumbling. Who holds the truth? Who decides what's remembered?

What This Chapter Offers: A vision of blockchain not as financial tool, but as moral infrastructure—a transparent, immutable, decentralised ledger of trust and testimony.

Why It Matters Now: In an age of erasure, disinformation, and distrust, sacred memory must be preserved in incorruptible form. Blockchain offers a surprising model.

> *"The past was erased, the erasure was forgotten, the lie became the truth."*
>
> — George Orwell, 1984

What if the most sacred thing about religion was never the ritual, but the record?

AI already shapes what we see, hear, and believe. But the real problem isn't AI itself—it's the creeping belief that data knows us better than we know ourselves. Algorithms become unblinking gods—not all-wise, but all-tracking. Blockchain mirrors that vigilance with one

crucial difference: it remembers without manipulation. Where AI curates and edits, a sacred ledger bears witness.

When Trust Is the Holiest Currency

To most, "blockchain" still conjures crypto hype, fraud, or speculative assets. But beneath the volatility lies a quieter revolution—one about trust. It answers an ancient spiritual question: Can we trust what's written?

Before scripture, there were ledgers: grain tallies pressed into Sumerian clay, priestly rolls in Egypt, monastic archives in medieval Europe. A ledger was never just a list; it was a collective memory of what mattered.

Religions have always honoured this instinct. The Torah is copied by hand with painstaking reverence. Christianity speaks of the Book of Life. Islam's Preserved Tablet holds the divine decree. Across traditions, memory was sacred—and written.

Blockchain reclaims this. No single priest or emperor holds the pen alone. The network shares it.

— It doesn't forget.

— It doesn't distort.

— It doesn't flatter.

In a digital world where truth is revised hourly, that's almost miraculous.

Why Faith Needs This

Faith begins where certainty ends. But trust in God often stumbles over distrust in institutions. Blockchain can't create belief, but it can protect its meaning.

Its properties—immutability, transparency, consensus—don't require shared doctrine, only a shared process. In this way, it mirrors the ethical clarity scripture once carried: a record that cannot be quietly rewritten.

Smart Contracts as Modern Covenant

Memory alone isn't enough. Spiritual life needs structure.

Smart contracts—code that executes promises—echo the form of ancient covenants. These could work alongside the covenants, liturgies, and practices already alive in churches and faith communities today:

If you rest, you'll be restored.

If you forgive, your heart will open.

If you give, your community will flourish.

Encoded intention could look like:

— A tithe automatically routed to mutual aid on feast days.

— A meditation log unlocking group participation.

— A covenant of care, signed and sealed across the network.

These are not decrees but chosen commitments—a contract not of guilt but gentle prompting: *You chose this. Stay true.*

The Risks—and the Reverence

Yes, blockchain has its own record of harm—scams, tribalism, greed—just as the history of religion includes seasons of crusades, corruption, and coercion. Sacred systems have always been fragile. The goal is not purity but possibility: a structure that can adapt while restoring trust where trust was lost.

Blockchain isn't sacred in itself, but it can be used reverently—to mark what matters and to make forgetting harder.

Memory is never neutral. It can convict or betray. The question is who holds it, and who may alter it. Orwell warned that the erasure of the past is the erasure of freedom. A sacred ledger resists both, guarding truth against sanctioned forgetting.

Data Isn't the Enemy of Devotion

We already live by ledgers: step counts, calendars, social feeds. We are measured constantly, yet rarely remembered.

What if the same tools kept what's worth keeping?

A gratitude ledger.

A forgiveness token.

A ritual contract—not for surveillance, but for continuity.

Stone tablets once seemed strange. So did printing presses. The sacred often takes an unfamiliar form.

Decentralisation as Reformation

History repeats: the printing press freed scripture from the pulpit, radio and TV carried it to the masses, the internet made it peer-to-peer.

Blockchain may free trust itself—not from faith, but from the vulnerabilities of monopoly—offering new ways to strengthen what faith communities already guard. It can encode covenant, preserve memory, and ritualise intention.

This doesn't pretend to be a substitute for God. Nor is it intended to replace the Church or the living traditions that have long carried sacred memory. It is simply one more vessel, built for this age, to help them endure. It's a way of protecting what God cares about: truth, trust, and community.

Distributed faith is durable faith.

A Closing Reflection

This chapter doesn't claim blockchain can save souls. It asks a different question:

What happens when we treat trust as sacred again—when our promises must be remembered, and carried?

A sacred ledger doesn't just record our faith; it shapes it, holding it steady against forgetting, revision, and quiet erasure.

If Orwell was right, then maybe the holiest act we can offer in the digital age is this:

To remember, together.

Chapter 8

The Protocol and the West

Can Faith Still Build a Civilisation?

Core Problem or Tension: The West did not emerge from neutrality. It was built on structured, enduring, self-correcting belief. But that scaffolding is crumbling. We've forgotten the covenantal core that once held law, learning, and liberty together.

What This Chapter Offers: A civilisational lens on D-Faith. This chapter explores how Western institutions—courts, cathedrals, charters—grew from theological assumptions, not mere politics. It proposes that for D-Faith to become more than a niche experiment, it must carry forward the moral architecture that once made the West exceptional.

Why It Matters Now: The West isn't collapsing from conquest, but from forgetting. As belief fades, the structures that bound freedom to responsibility erode too. D-Faith must offer a real alternative. Because if we don't rebuild moral architecture, the void won't stay empty—it will be filled by force or spectacle. The question isn't only whether faith can decentralise, it's whether anything lasting can still be built.

"The Christian ideal has not been tried and found wanting. It has been found difficult; and left untried."

— G.K. Chesterton

We don't usually think of civilisation as something built from belief. Yet, belief was infrastructure before roads or markets. Before governments, there were stories. Before laws, there was conscience.

What we now call *the West* didn't emerge from neutrality or chance. It grew from a particular way of believing—one that dignified the weak, anchored meaning in eternity, and wove moral structure into ritual, architecture, and learning.

> *"The Church gave the people a sense of purpose in life, a feeling of unity in a fragmented world, and a code of conduct more enduring than any law."*
>
> — Will Durant, The Story of Civilization

Christianity didn't just inspire awe. Through the Church, it built civilisations.

— Cathedrals. Charters. Universities.

— Hospitals without shareholders.

— A framework for both obedience and self-critique.

It gave people more than rules—a story they could inhabit, and institutions that could outlast the storytellers. Belief moved from the heart into stone, scroll, and custom. Conscience became culture.

The West as Exception

The West's distinctiveness was never about supremacy—it was about structure. For all its failings, it was the only civilisation we know that protected the individual conscience at scale while permitting open critique of its own foundations.

> *"To live in a Western country is to live in a society still utterly saturated by Christian concepts and assumptions."*
>
> — Tom Holland, Dominion

It built into its systems the possibility of repentance, allowed heresy to become reformation, and made space for the soul to wrestle in public.

No other civilisation quite produced that combination: liberty, law, science, and spirit—structured not for stasis but for survival through change. Even this book—its questions and provocations—would not have been possible under the caliphate, in revolutionary Iran, or dynastic China. The West was flawed, but it was singular.

The Fragile Retreat of Meaning

Today, belief retreats into privacy, meaning is commodified, and moral confidence is met with suspicion. Yet the ache does not vanish.

People still long for structure, trust, and something durable enough to hold life together, not just alone. D-Faith didn't rise from dominance but from the recognition of decay that the statistics reveal. It inherits no power. It begins where trust has been weakened—and seeks to build alongside and in service to living traditions.

This is a different kind of genesis: starting where institutions are brittle, and trust must be earned again, slowly, transparently.

Can D-Faith Help Strengthen What Christianity Built?

This is the test. Can decentralised faith do more than decentralise? Can it build? More accurate still, can it help restore belief in the West?

It will need more than technology. It will need covenant—a story worth transmitting, a structure worth trusting, and a moral logic that endures—even without enforcement.

In the past, Christianity achieved this through a deeply local and globally connected network. Parish churches and monasteries acted as redundant storage nodes—each holding the whole story, each capable of re-seeding it elsewhere if one fell. In a decentralised system, distributed storage layers such as IPFS or Filecoin could serve a similar role,

ensuring that sacred texts, communal decisions, and cultural memory cannot be erased by the failure or capture of a single node.

Doctrinal stewardship was never fully centralised; early church councils brought bishops from different regions together to deliberate, sometimes disagree, and maintain communion. Modern equivalents could be multi-stakeholder governance models—smart-contract frameworks where no single authority can alter core covenants without broad consensus, yet decisions can still be made.

Transmission across generations was once an embodied practice: scripture copied by hand, hymns taught by repetition, rituals embedded in the calendar. Immutable yet forkable record layers could carry that same durability today, preserving the original lineage even as local communities adapt its form.

Just as the church survived schisms, plagues, and political upheaval, decentralised networks are designed to withstand "partitions"—periods when parts of the network lose contact—and then resynchronise without data loss. The resilience of faith may one day rely on similar principles: that even under stress, the record remains whole, and trust can be rebuilt.

It must do what genuine faith has always done: shape souls, anchor communities, and survive its own contradictions. Its goal is not to replicate Christendom but to help remember and reinforce what once made civilisation coherent—and what will once again.

D-Faith will not endure because it is new. It will endure only if it dares what the West once dared—to build belief into something challenging, something lasting, something tried.

Chesterton would undoubtedly approve.

If it succeeds at all, it will be because it works in concert with the enduring witness of the Church and the communities that have carried faith through centuries of trial and change.

Chapter 9

From Rome to Reformation to Root Layer

Core Problem or Tension: The history of faith has swung like a pendulum between centralisation and fragmentation. Institutional religion brought order but also corruption; reform brought renewal but also disunity. Can faith adapt to digital disruption without ditching its ancient foundations?

What This Chapter Offers: Looking at Rome, Reformation, Enlightenment, and Modernity—culminating in a proposal for the next phase: a decentralised, incorruptible foundation for shared spiritual life. It introduces the metaphor of the "root layer," drawn from blockchain, as a blueprint for building spiritual systems that preserve trust, resist monopoly, and invite participation.

Why It Matters Now: The hunger for transcendence persists, but our frameworks are not serving. By revisiting the evolutionary arc of faith through the lens of systems design, this chapter lays the groundwork for reimagining sacred structure and speaks to modern minds without betraying ancient longings.

> "Every revolution is a restoration. Every reform is a recall to beginnings."
>
> — G.K. Chesterton

It's easy to imagine faith as static—passed down intact, bound in tradition, untouched by time. But history tells a more complex story. Faith doesn't vanish when institutions break down; it shifts shape. The longing for meaning remains, but how we carry it together changes.

Belief thrives by adapting. And the structures that hold it have always evolved with the times.

Rome: Faith as Structure and Sovereignty

For centuries, the Roman Catholic Church was more than a spiritual guide. It governed, preserved order, and guarded the metaphysical boundaries of truth. Doctrine was centralised. Sacraments mediated by clergy. Scripture read aloud but not freely studied. It helped build Europe's spine—but in some eras became deeply intertwined with empire.

Its moral clarity offered stability in a fractured world, but at the cost of control. Those who questioned doctrine had few options. Truth was not discerned in community—it was issued from above.

As historian Paul Johnson observed, the Church became an institution that "absorbed more than it released." Faith had, in that moment, taken on the form of a fortress—and fortresses, in time, can crack.

The Reformation: Faith as Protest

Luther never set out to fracture the Church. But in 1517, his hammer struck more than wood—it struck conscience. The printing press turned a private protest into a public revolution.

Interpretation no longer belonged solely to the priesthood. Scripture could be read, translated, and debated. Faith became personal, portable, and—often—polarised.

As Diarmaid MacCulloch noted, "What had once been one Church became a hundred." Protest fractured into proliferation. The Bible became more widely accessible—though often at the cost of shared consensus.

Faith had escaped control, but it had not escaped conflict.

> *"All the life and power of true religion consist in the inward and full persuasion of the mind; and faith is not faith without believing."*
> —John Locke, A Letter Concerning Toleration (1689)

This shift broadened freedom and made space for difference. But it also moved faith from the centre of public life to the margins. Religion became a lifestyle: browsable, personalised, compartmentalised.

We gained tolerance, but lost communion.

Modernity and the Silent Collapse

By the late 20th century, the outer forms of faith remained, but many were hollow. Churches stood, yet pews emptied. Rituals survived, but roots were shallow. Clergy once carried moral authority; now they competed with columnists and influencers.

And still, the ache persisted. The sacred didn't vanish—it migrated into politics, therapy, branding, and wellness. Francis Fukuyama observed that the longing for transcendence "has not disappeared—it has simply migrated."

We traded doctrine for discourse, myth for media, scripture for feeds. The need for spiritual architecture never left—it simply became harder to find.

The Root Layer: Toward a Decentralised Faith

So we arrive here.

What if faith had a root layer—incorruptible, participatory, transparent? It is not owned by any institution or altered in unseen corridors, but it is kept in common: visible, verifiable, and voluntary.

In blockchain terms, the root layer is the base protocol—unchangeable by one, requiring consensus to evolve. It secures memory through agreement alone.

Tradition need not be abandoned; it can be carried forward—open to contribution and resilient enough to grow. D-Faith isn't about escaping from the past but helping to preserve what is worth keeping—giving it a structure that can endure alongside the Church and other living traditions.

We've Been Here Before

The printing press was a proto-blockchain. It broke the monopoly on knowledge. Luther's tracts went viral. Tyndale's Bible was a fork of sacred code. Reformers wrote in ink what had been locked in Latin.

Now, the tools are stronger. We can share not only texts, but trust itself.

History leaves clues: when faith is absorbed into empire, it hardens and decays; when it breaks free through protest, it often splinters into factions. Transparent code could sustain it through both.

The Beginning Is Not the End

Most of us inherit faith like old furniture—heavy with meaning and awkward in modern rooms. We respect it, wrestle with it, and sometimes walk away from it.

Yet the instinct remains: to orient ourselves toward something higher, lasting, shared.

What we long for isn't nostalgia—it's rootedness. A structure strong enough to hold belief, even in doubt. A system that remembers what matters when everything else forgets.

Not just a new layer—

a root layer.

A return to the beginning—by way of the future.

If such a root layer is to last, it will need to stand in harmony with the Church that first carried these truths—strengthening the same witness in a form fit for the digital age.

Addendum: Historical–Technical Parallels for a Root Layer

The Church once built its "root layer" through networks of monasteries, parish churches, and travelling clergy—each a full copy of the faith's essential texts, rites, and memory. This redundancy meant that if one community fell, the whole was not lost. In a decentralised system, content-addressable storage like IPFS or Arweave serves the same purpose: every node carries the complete record and can restore the whole if part of the network is compromised.

When disputes arose—at Nicaea, Chalcedon, or Trent—the process resembled a multi-signature governance model: no single bishop could alter the creed, but consensus across many jurisdictions could adapt it. Similarly, doctrinal schisms are the historical equivalent of branching in Git: communities diverge in practice or belief while retaining an immutable shared ancestry.

Faith spread through replication—pilgrim routes, trade caravans, and local storytellers acted like peer-to-peer seeders, carrying the code of belief into new contexts. A modern root layer can replicate this organic propagation, not by control from the centre, but by ensuring every participant holds—and can transmit—the whole.

Interlude I: The Ever Hopeful Gardener

On Rebooting Eden, One Fork at a Time

> *"Nothing is ever enough. I couldn't create if it was. And now I must try it all again."*
>
> — "Him", Mother! (2017)

What if God isn't the unmoved mover, but the ever-hopeful re-maker? What if Eden wasn't the final plan, but the first prototype—a glimpse of harmony, knowing it wouldn't hold?

If God had wanted flawless obedience, He could have hard-coded it. But He didn't. He gave us freedom—and risked everything on how we'd respond.

And when we fail, He doesn't abandon the work. He starts again.

After Eden, He clothes us. After the flood, He offers covenant. After Babel, He lets us scatter—and later restores language at Pentecost, not through power, but presence. When law fails to transform, He sends not a rulebook, but a person—Jesus, with a towel in His hand.

Each divine restart moves us closer to communion, not control. God refines by remaining. Hope, not perfection, seems to be His strategy.

That same vision surfaces in art. In Darren Aronofsky's *Mother!* (2017), a godlike figure builds a world of beauty, watches it descend into chaos, and—heartbroken—begins again, not out of cynicism, but with quiet hope. It's uncomfortable to watch. But maybe faith is like that too: the courage to begin again, knowing it might break.

Could D-Faith be another such iteration? Not a replacement for the Church, but a continuation of that same sacred instinct—working alongside it to rebuild trust after collapse.

History shows this widening of participation: from temples to homes, from priests to people, from tablets of stone to truth written on hearts—without discarding the sacred communities that have carried that truth forward. Each reformation has loosened control and widened participation.

D-Faith doesn't claim flawlessness. But it offers something God seems to honour: freedom with accountability. It is a protocol built not on hierarchy but on traceable trust.

You may disagree. But let it be visible. Let others build from what you began. Be transparent in love.

No thrones. No walls. Just a ledger, a light, and the will to try again.

If it works at all, it will be because it shines alongside the enduring light of the Church, adding another lamp to the same house of faith.

Q: Didn't Christianity and other faith movements begin with small, decentralised groups? Wasn't it more authentic then?

A: Yes. Christianity began in homes, catacombs, and public squares, not in temples or state halls—among small groups sharing meals, stories, and risk. The early church had no central authority or branding, but it did have presence, conviction, and community. Protestant movements like the Baptists, Methodists, and Anabaptists also began this way—grassroots, peer-led, and conscience-driven. Of course, these movements had conflict and imperfection—but they pulsed with spiritual vitality and moral urgency. Far from rewriting history, the D-Faith model doesn't break with tradition; if anything, it mirrors the Church's earliest shape and spirit. Not to recreate the past, but to recover what made faith powerful.

And it seeks to do so in a way that strengthens the Church's continuing mission today.□

For a deeper exploration, *read "When It Was Small, It Was Alive" in the Bonus Materials.*

PART II: VISION & ARCHITECTURE

The D-Faith Protocol

"For where two or three are gathered in my name, there am I among them."

—Matthew 18:20

Chapter 10

Trust Without Priests

Rebuilding Spiritual Credibility Without Hierarchy

Core Problem or Tension: Faith traditions have long relied on intermediaries—priests, bishops, elders—to guard, interpret, and dispense spiritual authority. But centralised trust has proven fragile, vulnerable to corruption, exclusion and abuse. As institutional faith declines, a question emerges: Can trust in the sacred be rebuilt—without gatekeepers?

What This Chapter Offers: A vision of trust that doesn't require a gatekeeper. Drawing from both theology and decentralised systems, it introduces the idea of spiritual verification without hierarchy—trust distributed through shared rituals, code, and community.

Why It Matters Now: As institutional trust collapses across religion, government, and media, people seek new ways to anchor truth and accountability. This chapter shows how D-Faith can distribute responsibility without diluting reverence.

> *"I defy the Pope and all his laws. If God spare my life... I will cause a boy that driveth the plough to know more of the Scripture than thou dost."*
>
> — William Tyndale

In pre-literate societies, priests preserved sacred knowledge. But stewardship hardened into monopoly. Clerical classes gained wealth and influence—often becoming the very powers they once restrained.

Martin Luther opposed indulgences, yes, but also the idea that the laity could not understand Scripture. Early Gnostics were feared not just for their doctrine, but for bypassing the authorised path to God.

In economics, a bottleneck is a point of control: power flows one way; scrutiny doesn't return. Shoshana Zuboff, in *The Age of Surveillance Capitalism* (2019), warns that asymmetrical knowledge creates asymmetrical power. In some eras, aspects of the priesthood functioned like an early form of spiritual record-keeping—confessions gathered privately, interpreted within a framework of sanctioned authority.

Mystics and reformers were often cast out not for heresy but for independence, resulting in a loss of spiritual agency.

The Web as Revelation

The internet shattered that monopoly. Today, a seeker can explore the Dead Sea Scrolls, Buddhist sutras, and Sufi poetry without ever stepping inside a temple. Access abounds. Yet many still feel spiritually unanchored.

Like Bitcoin's assault on the global financial system, the web has opened faith to the public. But access alone doesn't create community. Without structure, belief drifts.

D-Faith doesn't discard wisdom—it makes it visible, verifiable, and voluntarily engaged.

Distributed Belief

Imagine a trust layer where:

— No one alters sacred principles alone
— Every contributor has a voice
— Rituals evolve through participation
— Identities are verified, but not centralised

This isn't theory. Web3 communities already work like this. Disputes lead to forks, not excommunications. Ethereum itself forked after crisis—and both versions survived.

D-Faith could offer the same resilience: forked traditions without erasure. As Iain McGilchrist notes in *The Master and His Emissary* (2010), we've overprivileged left-brain systems—hierarchy, control, decree. D-Faith proposes a right-brain alternative: relational, integrative, emergent.

From Clergy to Curators

If priests are no longer gatekeepers, who offers guidance?

Deuteronomy 19:15 insists that truth be confirmed "by the mouth of two or three witnesses"—a plural, participatory model.

D-Faith recovers this. It complements ordination with reputation—placing visible integrity alongside formal roles, allowing leadership to be both recognised and earned over time. This idea will be developed further in the Interpreter Layer, but its roots lie in trust earned in public view.

Is There Still a Place for Wisdom?

Yes—but not as a monopoly.

D-Faith resists consolidation by design:

— No central gatekeeper

— Transparency by default

— Forkable frameworks

— Influence based on trust, not title

As Phyllis Tickle wrote in *The Great Emergence* (2008), we are witnessing a "once-in-500-years" shift in authority, moving "from the pulpit to the circle." Leadership remains, but it is distributed.

Sacred Without Secrecy

Mystery invites reverence. Secrecy demands control. D-Faith treats transparency as sacred. Every theological claim is:

— Signed
— Timestamped
— Open-sourced

Disagreement means a fork, logged and visible. Like GitHub, strength grows through adoption, not by decree.

Guardrails Without Gatekeepers

What protects the sacred in such a system?

In blockchain, bad actors are exposed. Consensus replaces command, peer review replaces censorship, and reputation replaces hierarchy. As Rachel Botsman puts it in *Who Can You Trust?* (2017), we are entering an era of "distributed trust"—a new architecture for one of humanity's oldest needs.

Examples Emerging Now

The seeds are already here:

— Sacred Design Lab: open spiritual design
— Gitcoin DAOs: collective values in action
— Decentralised ID: new models for spiritual identity

Even the Vatican now experiments with lay consultation.

Together, these point to a movement toward open, self-governed spiritual life—one that isn't disorder, but renewal, freely embraced.

A Trust Structure That Doesn't Require Perfection

Traditional hierarchies often collapse under scandal because they are built to conceal it. D-Faith assumes imperfection and builds around it.

Reputation trails, transparent audits, forkable corrections—no one owns a belief, but everyone contributes to its memory. Leadership isn't absent; it's redistributed.

As Tyndale dreamed, the sacred may yet belong to the ploughboy—not by revolt, but through a system that moves at the speed of truth. An unstoppable, iridescent protocol built on light.

Postscript: When the Gatekeepers Panic

Every system resists what it cannot control—especially when it feels obsolete.

D-Faith doesn't seek to dismantle religion. It works alongside it, offering a parallel path for those outside the structures that have traditionally mediated access to God. No franchises. No toll booths. No permission slips. For some, that's the deepest threat of all.

For centuries, Church and State defined spiritual legitimacy—who could speak, what counted as sacred, which rituals bestowed belonging. Often, this came from sincere conviction. In an age before mass literacy or networks, intermediaries were necessary. Many still serve faithfully, with courage and sacrifice. The Church continues to carry the gospel faithfully in countless contexts, and D-Faith is not a replacement for that witness but a tool that can help protect and extend it in new ways. But D-Faith begins from a different premise: that access to God should never require permission, that spiritual truth is not proprietary, and that belonging does not depend on bureaucracy.

Pushback may not look like persecution. It may look like branding. Institutions may co-opt the language of decentralisation while keeping control. As governments mimic crypto with centralised currencies, faith organisations may launch "open" platforms that remain tightly managed.

As Rachel Botsman notes in *Who Can You Trust?*, distributed trust reshapes power—shifting it away from authority and toward architecture.

That's where D-Faith is strongest. It doesn't rely on charisma or protection. It is antifragile by design, drawing strength from friction. It allows forks rather than schisms, preserves transparent memory instead of managed history, depends on no leader who can be exiled and no node that can be shut down—reputation through visible action rather than inheritance.

Far from being a rebellion, it's a refuge for those whose longing has outgrown containment. And in time, some who first resisted may return—not because they have lost their faith, but because they aspire to more, and the gate no longer fits the size of their soul.

What D-Faith challenges is not truth, or love, or God—but the illusion that these can be owned, rather than stewarded as widely as humanly possible.

How Power Closes the Circle

Every system drifts toward centralisation. Leaders cluster. Decisions narrow. The few speak for the many. If nothing resists, the circle closes.

Six Ways to Keep It Open

1. **Forkable:** Let anyone take it and keep going.
2. **Public Record:** No secret history.
3. **Shared Keys:** No single gatekeeper.
4. **Rotate Roles:** Power should move.
5. **Low Gate:** Easy to join, easy to contribute.
6. **Celebrate Givers:** Reward sharing, not hoarding.

Chapter 11

The Interpreter Layer

— Replacing the Priest Without Replacing the Mystery

Core Problem or Tension: As people face grief, complexity, and contradiction, they reach for meaning—and interpretation begins. For millennia, power pooled where meaning was made. Even reformers rebuilt authority in their own image. How do we honour the sacred need for interpretation without falling back into control?

What This Chapter Offers: The *Interpreter Layer*—designed to meet this timeless need for discernment without replicating the power structures that too often distort it. We explore how decentralised, auditable, and AI-assisted interpretation might function. Inviting conscience rather than bypassing it.

Why It Matters Now: Modern spiritual seekers are not immune to the same risks of over-dependence, distortion, and passive consumption. As AI grows more persuasive the temptation to outsource spiritual reflection will only increase. We must design an interpretive system that *respects mystery, invites participation, and leaves final discernment to the soul.*

"My interpretation can only be as inerrant as I am, and that's good to keep in mind."

— Rachel Held Evans, Evolving in Monkey Town

The Eternal Struggle with Interpretation

Every tradition has faced it: meaning is not self-evident. Texts persist, but life evolves. Somewhere between revelation and routine, someone must interpret.

For centuries, clergy and scholars performed that task. At first, they offered guidance; in some contexts, guidance gradually hardened into rule. Interpretation could become permission—and permission often came from above.

Why Humans Reach for Interpreters

Interpretation is costly. It demands patience, grappling with contradiction, and deep reflection. As Daniel Kahneman and others have shown, the mind prefers shortcuts—not out of laziness, but because complexity is exhausting.

In matters of death, shame, justice, and meaning—where we cannot control the outcome—we at least strive for confidence. Priesthoods flourished because they answered the plea: *Tell me what this means, so I don't have to walk alone.*

Today, many turn to algorithms with the same longing. The instinct remains. Only the interface has changed.

D-Faith's Paradox

D-Faith avoids centralised hierarchy, punitive enforcement, and exclusive claims to truth, while honouring the wisdom that traditional interpretive roles have carried. But it still recognises the need that the priesthood once satisfied: the desire to *understand*.

So, how do we guide without control? Interpret without domination?

The Interpreter Layer

Enter the Interpreter Layer—a decentralised memory engine designed to support, not dictate. Think of it as a theological version-control system. It doesn't respond with "Thus saith the Lord," but with data, context, and transparency:

"In similar cases, 70% of nodes chose this path. Others diverged. Here are their reasons."

"Here are three reflections from contributors you follow—drawn from different traditions. Want to add your own?"

It's less like an explanation and more like a conversation.

Yes, It May Be AI—But Distributed and Transparent

The Interpreter Layer could run on decentralised AI systems like SingularityNet or Bittensor. It might:

—Train only on witnessed, opt-in reflections

— Offer traceable lineage for every response

— Support forked versions and interpretive "subcultures" (poetic, legalist, contemplative)

— Say "*I don't know*" when reverence is the proper reply

The Role of Conscience and Community

Every interpretive suggestion would include:

A traceable contributor trail (anonymous or pseudonymous)

— A version history

— The option to refine or fork

Interpretation is not outsourced to a licenced third party—it is shared. The Layer always listens before it speaks.

What AI Interpretation Is Not

It is not divine. It cannot punish. It cannot replace awe.

It fails its purpose if it ever claims to replace God's voice or the discernment of the Church. That safeguard would be inscribed in the Genesis Document itself.

Use Cases in Daily Life

Imagine a parent facing a difficult choice—whether to withdraw her child from a school that is academically strong but spiritually corrosive. In the Interpreter Layer, she requests input from across the network. Within hours, she receives three reflections: one rooted in Scripture, one in secular child development research, and one from a trauma-informed pastoral counsellor. Each entry is linked to its contributor's trust history and citations. She can see which perspectives have been affirmed by others she follows and how often each source has revised their own positions.

Or picture a small D-Faith node designing a new coming-of-age ritual. They search the Interpreter Layer for "rites of passage" and pull up examples: a South African confirmation liturgy, a Zen Buddhist *Jukai* ceremony, and a modern Quaker welcome. They can fork one, adapt it, and push the updated version back into the shared memory, complete with their rationale for each change.

A former believer might return and anonymously offer a story. The community bears witness, and the story enters the shared memory chain.

This is spiritual guidance that listens first.

Guardrails Against a New Priesthood

To avoid rebuilding the very problem it seeks to solve, the Interpreter Layer includes:

Peer verification
— Open review rituals
— On-chain logging of misuses
— Transparent correction

The Preservation of Mystery

Some questions are not meant to be resolved. The Interpreter Layer can pause. This one leaves space.

It approaches quietly, not forcefully.

It offers perspectives, not fixed answers.

Interpretation becomes a shared process—woven from many memories and insights, rather than set by a single voice.

Rachel Held Evans reminded us: "My interpretation can only be as inerrant as I am."

The Interpreter Layer takes that humility and builds it into the code. It assumes no one sees the whole picture, but that together—through visible, accountable, and diverse interpretation—we might see more.

It does not ask for blind trust. It asks us to walk in good faith—aware of our limits, but unwilling to have those limits set for us.

This interpretive approach is available for those who cannot, or choose not to, seek the guidance of pastors, priests, or theologians. It extends their work into a transparent, participatory layer—helping safeguard and share their wisdom across a wider network.

Technical Supplement: Interpreter Layer

For the Interpreter Layer to guide without ruling, it must embody the same decentralised principles as D-Faith itself. That means:

1. Forked interpretive histories

Just as code repositories can branch, interpretive threads could fork without erasing their origin. A poetic reading of a text might evolve separately from a legalist one, yet both would retain a shared lineage, making it possible to trace how understanding diverged over time.

2. Opt-in training datasets

Only reflections that have been consciously contributed and cryptographically signed are used for training. This ensures that the "voice" of the Interpreter Layer comes entirely from willing participants, not scraped or co-opted material.

3. Contributorship as consensus

A change to interpretive framing—such as redefining a term or re-weighting a tradition—would require a threshold of agreement among active contributors, verified by multi-signature governance. No single node could steer meaning unilaterally—mirroring the conciliar traditions of the Church, where consensus has long been a safeguard of truth.

4. Preserving 'I don't know'

The system could be programmed with humility triggers—thresholds where interpretive confidence falls below a set level, prompting the Layer to say *This one requires silence* rather than fabricating certainty. These thresholds are adjustable by community governance.

5. Anchored version control

Whether accepted or ignored, every suggestion is stored with an immutable timestamp and contributor signature. This builds a visible memory of how a community wrestled with questions over time—an unbroken audit trail of conscience.

In combination, these mechanics give the Interpreter Layer not only resilience against abuse but also a living archive of interpretive diversity—its strength lies in its plurality, not its unanimity.

Chapter 12

Coding Sacred Systems

Core Problem or Tension: Our technologies encode values, yet those values are often unconscious or utilitarian. The systems we build—algorithms, platforms, contracts—shape human behavior, but rarely with sacred intention.

What This Chapter Offers: This chapter explores how technology, especially decentralised infrastructure like smart contracts and consensus protocols, can be designed with spiritual and moral principles. It asks: what if code was covenantal? What if systems could encode reverence, trust, and alignment?

Why It Matters Now: As technology continues to intermediate nearly every aspect of life, the risk grows that we build efficient tools for a spiritually empty world. This chapter offers a blueprint for building systems that not only function, but nourish.

> *"There is no unsacred place; there are only sacred places and desecrated places."*
>
> — Wendell Berry

Everything can be sacred—or desecrated. Technology too.

What if covenant could also live in code—not only in scrolls or stone, not only recited in ritual or guided by clergy, but embedded into the systems through which we live, decide, and belong?

Code as Covenant

Code isn't neutral. It shapes behaviour. A smart contract doesn't request agreement—it executes. *If this, then that.* No debate. No appeal.

In this way, code resembles divine speech—abstract yet governing. It performs rather than persuades. Could it also ground a shared ethical life?

Think of it as a moral operating system—not a new religion, but digital scaffolding for conscience that can serve and strengthen the faith traditions already guiding communities today.

The Moral OS

We already have examples:

— *Wikipedia* encodes neutrality.

— *Bitcoin* encodes scarcity and censorship resistance.

— *The Montessori Method* encodes autonomy in design.

D-Faith could encode its own:

— Transparent protocols that resist corruption.

— Rituals immune to personality cults.

— Covenants with version control—truth that evolves in daylight.

As Lawrence Lessig wrote, *"Code is law."* For D-Faith, perhaps code becomes covenant.

The Problem of Rigidity

Pure code is unforgiving. It cannot show mercy. It cannot grow.

That's why grace must be structural:

— **Versioning:** to show change over time

— **Reconciliation tokens:** witnessed, symbolic repair

— **Emergency exits:** for systemic harm

— **Ritual audits:** because what's sacred must also stay alive

Religious traditions have long done this:

— The Talmud revises through argument

— Christian reformations rearticulated and, in some cases, reshaped the canon

— Islamic fiqh adapts law to context and conscience

Flexibility isn't moral compromise—it's moral maturity.

We Already Live Inside These Experiments

Our digital spaces already run on moral operating systems:

— *GitHub* governs through rules and pull requests

— *Airbnb* builds trust through ratings, not contracts

— *DAOs* encode values via transparent votes

Faith is adapting too:

— *Unitarian Universalists* vote on ethical declarations.

— *Confessional apps* encode intimacy (e.g., Confessit).

— *Digital synods* invite open consultation.

These aren't novelties. They're signals: the sacred is reformatting.

Covenant 2.0

Old covenants were sealed with sacrifice. New ones may be sealed with hashes. But the longing beneath is timeless:

To be seen.

To be safe.

To act in good faith.

To grow—without erasure.

Imagine a small interfaith community spread across five countries. They draft a shared covenant—a commitment to monthly acts of hospitality—recorded as a *commitment hash* on the D-Faith chain. The text of the covenant lives in distributed storage; each member's signature is cryptographically linked.

Every month, each participant logs a short encrypted note when they've kept the practice: "*Hosted a meal for a neighbour,*" "*Welcomed a newcomer at the market,*" "*Shared tea with someone grieving.*" The zero-knowledge layer verifies that the action meets the covenant's criteria without revealing the private details.

When one member suggests adding a seasonal focus—hospitality to refugees in winter—the group proposes an update. It can only be ratified during their *seasonal consensus window*, so the idea circulates for weeks, gathering comments and refinements before the change is adopted.

Five years on, the moral audit trail shows not just that the covenant has endured, but *how* it has evolved—every amendment tagged with its rationale, every fork preserved so no memory is lost.

A moral OS won't be perfect. But it can be sincere, transparent, and participatory—built to carry not only memory and mercy, but reverence. A covenant might begin as a *commitment hash*—a timestamped signature of a promise, light enough to store forever, yet able to keep its private details sealed unless consented. Some would run as *ritual state machines*, moving forward only when agreed-upon acts—like reconciliation—are completed.

Changes could be tracked with *context tags*, showing the new version and why it changed. Ratifications might happen in *seasonal consensus windows*—fixed moments in the year that slow down edits and make them deliberate. Over time, a *moral audit trail* would emerge: not only what changed, but why—a living commentary as much as a record.

As code begins to shape how we live, it will also shape what we hold sacred—or what we allow to be desecrated. That is why covenant must be intentional: abandoning control and obedience for commitment and trust. As Berry reminds us, there is no neutral ground—only what we choose to make sacred and what we allow to be lost.

In this vision, code becomes another servant of the covenant—extending the Church's or any tradition's role in shaping sacred life into

a realm where memory, mercy, and reverence can be sustained in new ways.

Q: *What did Satoshi actually create?*

A: Before the headlines, before the hype, there was just a document. Nine pages of careful thought. A small piece of open-source code. And one silent block, stamped with a line from the news.

There were no executives. No investors. No product launch. Just a modest offering: a way of recording trust that didn't rely on authority. A system that asked nothing of you except to understand it—and, if moved, to take part in building it.

It was born in obscurity, refined through dialogue, and kept alive by people who believed that honesty could be written into code. Most earned nothing for their efforts. Some are still anonymous. Even the one called Satoshi left without fanfare—and has yet to take a single coin.

Yes, it may have been about inventing money. But it also proved something greater: that belief, freely shared and humbly maintained, can still change the world.

Maybe that's the real blueprint worth following.

For a deeper exploration, read "What Did Satoshi Actually Create?" in the Bonus Materials.

Chapter 13

The Sacred Record

Source and Chain in a Decentralised Faith

Core Problem or Tension: How do we preserve what's sacred—without surrendering it to control? Religions have long used hierarchy to safeguard memory. Yet when memory is left entirely to individuals, it fragments and fades. The tension is clear: Can we build shared spiritual memory without gatekeepers?

What This Chapter Offers: This chapter explores the idea of a decentralised spiritual record. Inspired by blockchain, It asks how we might witness to faith without relying on authority, and how memory can be distributed yet trustworthy. Drawing on both technological metaphors and spiritual traditions, it introduces the idea of a Sacred Ledger: a way to encode moral presence without institutional oversight, and to preserve meaning across time without requiring uniformity.

Why It Matters Now: Who curates the story when no one's in charge? Without memory, we lose coherence. Without trust, we lose each other. A transparent, incorruptible record of spiritual life may be the key to continuity in an era of collapse.

"Blockchain allows us to redefine trust and enable peer□-to□peer transactions without intermediaries."

—□Vitalik Buterin

Every lasting tradition depends on memory—yet memory, left unguarded, can be rewritten by power.

For the Abrahamic faiths, memory was sacred: a breath into clay, a whisper in a cave, a voice in a bush. Enlightenment humanism placed its trust in reason and text. Blockchain anchors trust in a protocol—Satoshi's nine-page white paper that seeded a trillion-dollar ecosystem without needing anyone's permission.

Each began with a record.

Not because the divine forgets—

But because we do.

The Sacred Record

D-Faith's Sacred Record doesn't replace scripture or the Church's role in preserving it; it reflects presence. It holds moments of conscience, turning points, and returns—a covenantal memory that doesn't require hierarchy to be holy. This is not intended to supplant the long tradition of sacred record-keeping in churches, monasteries, and archives, but to complement it with tools designed for a decentralised age.

Can You Confess to the Chain?

Confession was never meant as surveillance. It was sacred risk, a way to say, "*I turned back today.*"

In D-Faith, there is no booth or gatekeeper. Yet something of that grace remains. You might log:

— A moment of restraint, grief, or hope

— A symbol of conscience, sealed in privacy

— A timestamp of return—seen, but not explained

Like lighting a candle behind a veil, others see the glow, not the flame.

Picture a seasonal gratitude ritual shared by dozens of D-Faith nodes. At the end of each season, members log one encrypted act

> of gratitude—helping a neighbour, funding a need, or reconciling with someone estranged. Zero-knowledge proofs verify it as an act of gratitude without revealing its content.
> The record is timestamped, publicly verifiable, and permanently linked to that season's covenant. Over time, a visible pattern emerges—perhaps 80% participation in spring, 92% in autumn—without exposing individual actions. This data helps the community reflect honestly on its spiritual health, just as liturgical calendars once marked the pulse of shared devotion.□
> Because the Sacred Record is forkable, a node could create its own variation—a "justice ledger" for advocacy actions, or a "mercy ledger" for care work—while still inheriting the core format. Each fork preserves the shared lineage, ensuring that even local adaptations remain part of the collective memory.

In D-Faith, zero-knowledge proofs make this possible. They let you demonstrate that something happened without revealing what happened. A believer might commit a private act—fasting, reconciling, returning to a discipline—and log it as an encrypted entry in the Sacred Record. The blockchain confirms its authenticity and timestamp, while the zero-knowledge layer proves it matches a chosen category (e.g., "ritual kept," "promise renewed") without exposing the act itself.

It's like showing a sealed envelope stamped by a notary. Everyone can see the seal is genuine; no one opens the envelope. The Sacred Record stays honest without becoming surveillance—memory anchored in trust, without prying eyes.

With zero-knowledge proofs, you can prove consistency without revealing content. This isn't just theory—similar privacy-preserving systems are already trusted in high-stakes environments. Zcash uses them to enable anonymous yet verifiable financial transactions. The voting platform Helios has explored them to confirm election results without revealing individual ballots. In each case, trust is maintained because verification does not require exposure.

The proof that something sacred occurred—without handing it over to be managed, judged, or possessed—is itself part of the reverence.

Memory With Consent

The Sacred Record is never public by default. You decide what's recorded and who may witness it. There is no spiritual scorekeeping, no gamified virtue.

Vitalik Buterin imagined blockchain as trust without intermediaries. D-Faith extends that vision to trust with reverence—where sacred moments are remembered, not curated, or managed.

Because not every form of reflection or testimony requires a priest—though the Church's sacramental confession remains vital for many.

Some need a place to be kept.

And sometimes trust isn't built by control at all—

It's built by choosing to remember, together.

In this way, the Sacred Record can work alongside the living witness of the Church, extending its memory into new spaces while honouring the traditions that have kept it for centuries.

Q: *Is Anything Truly Private in a Decentralised Faith?*

A: In D-Faith, privacy is not an afterthought—it's foundational. Every entry is stored by the user—a vow, a reflection, a turning point. Some are encrypted for personal access only. Some are visible to a trusted circle. Others are written permanently into the chain, but never exposed without explicit permission.

Reputation forms through consistent action under a chosen pseudonym—not a legal name. The system doesn't demand trust through exposure; it allows trust to build through choice and control. People can be known, grow, and contribute without handing over their identity or history.

D-Faith doesn't monitor behaviour or mine data—just as the Church's safeguarding of confession rests on voluntary disclosure and trust. It records what's given, not what's taken. What you choose to store becomes part of a distributed memory—durable, incorruptible, and under your control, whether personal or shared.

It's a design intended to complement the Church's pastoral and sacramental settings—extending the space where conscience can be exercised freely and securely.

For a deeper exploration, read "Data Privacy" in the Bonus Materials.

Chapter 14

Can Faith Be Forked?

Diverging Viewpoints in a Decentralised Age

Core Problem or Tension: Religious institutions have long treated schism as failure. But in a decentralised world, divergence may be a sign of system vitality—not collapse.

What This Chapter Offers: A reframing of religious "forking" as a spiritual design feature, drawing from blockchain governance and religious history alike. This chapter focuses on technical design, governance implications, and system viability.

Why It Matters Now: As more people lose trust in centralised institutions, we need a model of faith that can evolve without fragmenting—and honor conscience without chaos.

> *"What we call the beginning is often the end. And to make an end is to make a beginning."*
>
> — T.S. Eliot

The sacred has never stood still.

Christianity was fractured into Catholic and Orthodox, then split again during the Reformation. Islam divided into Sunni and Shia. Buddhism diverged into Theravada and Mahayana.

These were not only political or cultural schisms—they were theological forks: disorganised, risky, and often necessary. And yet, belief didn't vanish. It adapted. It grew.

A fork, in code, doesn't erase what came before—it branches. Ethereum forked after a crisis. Bitcoin has forked many times. Some splinters thrive, others fade. But the protocol remains. Faith can work the same way.

Lessons from the Blockchain

Blockchains assume divergence. They're built for it. Nodes disagree, negotiate, and update—without collapse. Without the need for papal councils or decrees in this model (though those remain vital within the Church's own governance) D-Faith relies on structure and transparency.

We already trust fork-resilient systems in high-stakes environments:

— The Linux operating system has hundreds of forks, yet its shared kernel keeps it coherent.

— Wikipedia's open-edit model allows content forks, but its revision history preserves every prior version.

D-Faith applies the same principle to belief. It accepts that people already remix tradition: blending rituals, reinterpreting doctrine, stepping away from institutions while still longing for the sacred. The difference is that here, the forking is visible, ethical, and accountable.

In practice, every fork in D-Faith is anchored to the Genesis Document—a set of transcendent principles like love, conscience, truth, and reverence. Any node can propose a fork, but the new branch must include a public changelog explaining *why* the divergence exists and *what* it preserves. Forks that attract active contributors, consistent participation, and relational trust will naturally thrive; those without gravity fade into archival memory. The record of every fork remains accessible, so history can be rejoined without erasure.

Sacred Divergence vs. Doctrinal Chaos

Does everything dissolve without hierarchy? Not if we design wisely. In crypto, most forks fail—not by suppression but by irrelevance. They lack coherence, trust, or fruit.

D-Faith's root layer functions like TCP/IP for belief: it keeps the network interoperable even as branches grow in different directions.

In this way, D-Faith doesn't replace the stabilising role of the Church but offers a complementary space where conscience-led divergence can be recorded, remembered, and, where possible, reconciled.

Authority Without Centralisation

In decentralised faith, authority is earned, not bestowed by title or position. Any node—a person, group, or text—may contribute insight. Like GitHub for theology, you can fork, annotate, propose changes, and be recognised for your contributions—not only your position—while still drawing on the wisdom of existing Church traditions.

It's already happening: Celtic-inspired liturgies used in Anglican churches, Jewish Sabbath practices adapted by secular wellness groups, and digital-first communities co-creating seasonal rituals without a central bishop or board.

The Role of Conscience in Forking

Vaclav Havel called conscience "the compass of the soul." In D-Faith, it's also the governance layer. But conscience must be shaped—through listening, humility, and reflection. Not all divergence is wise. Not all reform is renewal.

The open-source world knows this well: not every fork improves the project; some are vanity exercises, others dead ends. The same discernment applies here.

Toward a Fork-Resilient Faith

Fork-resilient faith bends like evolution—anticipating divergence while keeping coherence from a shared source. In a world of institutional collapse and mass disillusionment, designing for pluralism may be the only viable way forward, not by suppressing difference, but by making space for divergent devotion.

If we can fork with memory and mercy, trusting a greater source, then Eliot was right: every end is a beginning. And sometimes, the sacred splits to survive.

If so, D-Faith—and the Church that has carried Christianity through the centuries—will not only survive, but may flourish together. It may be through divergence, not dogma, that we find our way back to each other.

Chapter 15

DAOs, Rituals, and Sacred Action

If code is the covenant, action is the liturgy

Core Problem or Tension: Traditional religions offered rituals that created meaning, memory, and moral formation. But in a decentralised world, how can shared sacred action persist?

What This Chapter Offers: A look at DAOs (Decentralised Autonomous Organisations) not just as governance tools, but as liturgical engines—spaces where community, ritual, and sacred intent can align through technology.

Why It Matters Now: Without shared rituals, faith becomes private and disembodied. This chapter shows how DAOs and other digital forms can host communal practices that encode value and foster belonging.

> "People don't just need to believe in something. They need to belong to something."
>
> — David Brooks

Brooks reminds us that belief isn't enough—we crave belonging, and rituals are how belonging becomes real.

Why Ritual Still Matters

Covenant is what we commit to. Liturgy is how we live it—repeatedly, together. If code encodes values, ritual enacts them. It's how belief moves from abstract to embodied.

Even in secular life, we reach for proto-rituals: lighting candles, pressing *send*, making a wish before cake. These small acts root meaning in the body.

Neuroscientist Pascal Boyer found that rituals "stick" because they engage the senses, community, and repetition. If belief is software, ritual is the interface. It trains attention, forms memory, and anchors identity. That's why religious and civic life—whether a Catholic mass or singing a national anthem—rely on ritual to turn ideas into identity.

What Are DAOs?

DAOs are online communities built to act with purpose, without a central leader. Shared rules are encoded in smart contracts, and decisions are made openly and together.

Think of them as a digital parallel to monasteries or congregations—different in form, without abbots, bishops, or pews, yet able to work alongside these existing communities. They already exist for climate action, artist collectives, and mutual aid[1].

So why not spiritual life?

In D-Faith, DAOs could:

— Share commitments to prayer or reflection.

— Pool resources for acts of compassion.

— Design new rituals together, shaped by consensus rather than decree.

---

1. I.e. (*KlimaDAO*, funding carbon offsets), artist collectives (*PleasrDAO*, co-owning culturally significant digital art), and mutual aid (*UkraineDAO*, raising humanitarian funds) and even spiritual exploration (**FaithDAO**, funding interfaith projects and sacred art).

These are proto-liturgical structures—ritual shaped by code rather than solely by clergy, and designed to complement the sacred forms already carried by faith traditions.

Rituals in a Decentralised Context

What might D-Faith rituals look like?

— A "Consensus Fast" before votes, to clarify intent

— Symbolic micro-donations—signals of gratitude

— Meditations in sync with block confirmations—a sacred rhythm tied to code

Or imagine a *Sabbath Lighting Network*: nodes worldwide record a simple on-chain signal each Friday at sunset when they light their candles. The act is private—the flame, the prayers, the faces stay unseen—but the network map glows with points of light, a shared moment across continents.

Or a *Ramadan Fast Tracker*: participants log daily fast completions with zero-knowledge proofs, proving faithfulness to the rhythm without revealing personal health data or private struggles. Communities could even pledge pooled donations unlocked when the fast cycle completes, tying ritual directly to tangible good.

Like open-source liturgy, these rituals are visible but not performative. They're not about scoring points or proving devotion—they're about showing up with sincerity, again and again.

The Power of Visibility

In traditional faiths, ritual was visible in pilgrimages, shared meals, and blessings. It made belief public—and continues to do so today.

Blockchain offers similar visibility—actions are recorded, traced, and remembered. The difference is control: in D-Faith, the participant chooses what's visible. Just as Zcash allows a transaction to be verified without revealing its details, a D-Faith ritual could be confirmed without exposing private meaning.

Challenges and Cautions

Ritual can harden into hierarchy. That's why D-Faith rituals must be:

— **Editable**: Versioned and improved

— **Inclusive**: Accessible across devices and abilities

— **Meaningful**: Never spiritual cosplay

Regular retrospectives—like Agile sprints—keep practice honest and alive.

Spiritual Prototypes

We're already experimenting:

— **Gitcoin**: Public funding as shared moral gesture

— **CabinDAO**: Seasonal gatherings meet digital governance

— **MetaCartel**: Calls feel like early house churches

Beyond blockchain: mutual aid pods that bless food; grief circles that livestream silence. These aren't gimmicks—they're signals of longing for presence, purpose, and sacred rhythm.

Moving Toward Sacred Action

DAOs and rituals let us enact belief, not just profess it. They turn habit into culture, culture into covenant. Sacredness isn't proven by sentiment, but by what we practice together.

In the end, belief without belonging dries out. Ritual becomes the rhythm that turns ideas into lived experience, especially when shared. DAOs and sacred protocols aren't just about consensus but communion. They give us ways to show up, contribute, and be witnessed.

Brooks was right: people don't just want to believe. They want to belong, not in theory, but through action. And when we move together, with intention and grace, we don't just preserve meaning. We create it—together.

And where these new forms emerge, they can sit alongside the Church's enduring rhythms—offering another way for the same sacred pulse to be felt across distance, while remaining connected to the wisdom of tradition.

Chapter 16

Nodes of Light:

Community Without Control

Core Problem or Tension: Traditional spiritual communities have often relied on hierarchy and control to ensure stability. How do we build authentic spiritual connection without that oversight? In a decentralised system of faith, where no institution enforces belonging, how do we rediscover the sacred bonds that hold us together?

What This Chapter Offers: This chapter proposes the idea of "nodes of light": spiritually aligned micro-communities that grow through trust, shared values, and lived ritual rather than organisational command. Drawing on ancient wisdom, modern networks, and experimental spiritual practices, it offers a model for belonging that is adaptive, human, and sacred.

Why It Matters Now: People still yearn for genuine connection rooted in meaning. But few new structures meet that need. This chapter outlines how decentralised communities—formed by consent, sustained by trust—can offer depth, accountability, and joy without the machinery of control.

"There is no power for change greater than a community discovering what it cares about."

— Margaret Wheatley

For centuries, much spiritual life has been centralised—guided by clergy, rooted in sacred buildings, and sometimes directed by distant authority.

D-Faith expands the focus from congregations alone to also include nodes—circles of trust that can work alongside established communities. A node might be a kitchen table, a group chat, or a grief circle. What matters is shared intention, not formal authority.

Henri Nouwen wrote, *"Community is the fruit of our capacity to make the interests of others more important than our own."* In this model, community isn't managed. It's lived into, through daily acts of care and presence.

Victor Turner called it *communitas*—raw, sacred connection that can't be programmed. We may stream sermons but miss sitting with others in shared silence, grief, or joy.

D-Faith must make space for that ache — through ritual, safety, and intimacy offered and received by choice.

The Technology of Trust

Blockchain can decentralise trust, but humans still need to be seen. In D-Faith, a node might show its values through visible action: generosity logs, consensus rituals, transparent departures.

Imagine a small bereavement node that keeps a *care ledger*: members commit to checking in weekly with anyone newly bereaved, logging the act on-chain without revealing details. Or imagine a justice-oriented node that records acts of advocacy—letters sent, protests attended, petitions signed—each one verified by two other members. These aren't virtue signals; they're proofs of presence.

Trust isn't automated. It's grown slowly through presence and participation.

Designing for the Soul

Faith doesn't depend solely on control; it thrives on coherence. You join a node because its values resonate. And if not, you fork.

Some groups will falter, others flourish. That's antifragility in action. Forests don't fear fallen trees—they grow through them.

Communities like the Bruderhof, Alcoholics Anonymous, and Torah study pods show what's already possible.

Meals, music, silence—these are the new protocols. In a D-Faith context, that might look like a monthly "shared table" ritual where every node hosts a meal on the same day, photographing only the empty table afterward to mark the gathering without intruding on the moment. Or it could be a cross-node "Night of Listening" where members from different geographies log on for an hour of silent presence, recorded only as a timestamp on the network.

No one owns these practices, but together, they help us belong again.

Shekhinah still arrives, wherever two or three gather. And whether that gathering is in a centuries-old cathedral or a kitchen table node, the same Spirit binds it to the long witness of the Church.

Chapter 17

Sacred Simplicity

Core Problem or Tension: Modern life is a blur of stimulation, velocity, and superficiality. Many long for a deeper rhythm but feel trapped in habits and systems that fragment rather than complete. The sacred feels distant not because it disappeared—but because it got crowded out.

What This Chapter Offers: This chapter invites a reorientation toward sacred simplicity—less minimalism, more intentionality. It draws on spiritual traditions like the Sabbath, monastic design, and moral UX to explore how we might encode awe, rhythm, and reverence into daily life. It bridges old wisdom with new tools, showing how simplicity can be a design principle for the soul.

Why It Matters Now: Overwhelm is the new baseline. Constant connectivity has collapsed boundaries between work and rest. Without simplicity, even faith becomes fragmented. Reclaiming sacred rhythm is not a nostalgic "nice-to-have"—it's both essential and urgent.

"It is not daily increase but daily decrease—hack away the unessential."

—Bruce Lee

What does it mean to live a good life, not just ethically or efficiently, but sacredly?

Sacred simplicity isn't minimalism. It's meaningful presence where we say no to distraction and yes to what matters. It provides a space where awe can land, where silence or a break in the usual rhythm of life, doesn't feel like it was forced into the diary, but enthusiastically embraced when it comes.

Abraham Joshua Heschel described the Sabbath—still faithfully kept in many Jewish and Christian communities—as "*a sanctuary in time.*" A weekly ceasefire with the world, it functions as spiritual infrastructure: a moral user interface that encodes rest, reverence, and memory.

Even in a digital faith network, sacredness can mean stepping away from the screen[1] . This could mean *screen sabbaths*—devices off from sunset Friday to sunset Saturday—or *relational rituals* like the "slow dinner" movement, where meals stretch for hours and phones stay out of sight. It could also mean using a pared-down version of D-Faith, with only essential features active, to create space for presence.

James Clear reminds us, *"Environment is the invisible hand that shapes human behavior."* Sacredness needs a setting to land in: a candle before dinner, a phone set aside, a pause before speaking.

Productivity fills time, and sacredness inhabits it. Shared meals, deep breaths, and lingering pauses aren't interruptions to faith; they are its rhythm.

Simplicity as Spiritual Resistance

In a culture that monetises attention, simplicity becomes an act of moral defiance. Wendell Berry wrote, *"We live in a world not made for us."* He names the discomfort many feel but can't quite articulate—a world optimised for profit, at the expense of presence. Sacred simplicity

1. Even in a digital faith network, sacredness may require closing the laptop, silencing the phone, and letting stillness whisper.

replies: *"Then let's make it a world worth inhabiting."* Not through grand gestures, but through ritual, rhythm, and slowness.

Small practices—gratitude before meals, phones in a basket, lighting a candle at dusk—aren't mere nostalgia, but living ceremony. They're rewiring the everyday patterns that we occupy on auto-pilot. Even secular thinkers like Cal Newport (*Deep Work*) and Tristan Harris (*Humane Tech*) point toward the same hunger: for rhythms that calm the nervous system, focus the mind, and offer meaning beyond productivity.

Imagine a quiet daily covenant:

— **Morning:** Experience wonder (watch sunrise, read sacred text, walk without headphones).

— **Midday:** Contribute (serve someone, work with care, share generously).

— **Dusk:** Reflect (review the day, note gratitude, close with stillness).

Not replacing doctrine—designing alongside it.

Many of these practices are already embedded in the Church's liturgical year, monastic hours, and communal life. Sacred simplicity in a decentralised context adopts similar patterns—it translates them for a scattered and digital world.

Designing for the Soul

Technology already decides what we notice, how we spend, and when we pause. D-Faith uses that same power to nudge us away from distraction and consumption toward reflection, connection, and shared meaning—what matters most.

A browser extension that prompts a breath every hour.

A wallet that flags spending at odds with your stated values.

A calendar that reserves time for stillness, the way it does for meetings.

This is UX as spiritual design—intention built into our daily interactions.

Simone Weil wrote, *"Attention, taken to its highest degree, is the same thing as prayer."* Sacred simplicity at its most effective will be a structure that sustains not only belief, but daily behaviours.

When many live this way—attentive, slowed, oriented—faith becomes less an effort and more a rhythm. When meaning no longer needs to be forced, it emerges naturally.

Because, as Bruce Lee taught, the path isn't in adding more. It's in removing what distracts from what's essential.

Sacred simplicity isn't about doing less. It's about repeatedly doing what matters—on purpose, with grace. Strip away the noise. What's left might just be holy.

And in whatever form it's practised—whether in a centuries-old sanctuary or a digital covenant—this rhythm draws from the same well the Church has kept flowing for generations.

Chapter 18

The Witness Layer:

Spiritual Proof-of-Work

Core Problem or Tension: In an age of disinformation and algorithmic manipulation, a pressing question emerges: Who do we trust; how do we know they tell the truth? A decentralised faith must reckon with the tension between openness and credibility. Without hierarchy, how is moral integrity verified? How do we distinguish between performative virtue and authenticity?

What This Chapter Offers: The "*witness layer*"—a human/spiritual analogue to blockchain's proof-of-work. Drawing from religious history, cryptographic principles, and lived moral action, it proposes a model where credibility is earned through perseverance. Where the most trustworthy voices are those whose lives have borne the cost of love. It asks: "*If no one is in charge, why believe anyone at all?*"

Why It Matters Now: In a post-truth culture, we're starved for proof. The witness layer offers an answer: a decentralised network of trust built on sacrifice, consistency, and humility. It's not about creating influencers—it's about building gravity.

"Your life as a Christian should make nonbelievers question their disbelief in God."

—Dietrich Bonhoeffer

Pilate's question—*What is truth?*—was never answered. He didn't wait.

Sacred traditions have always pointed in the same direction: not argument, but embodiment. The ones we trust are not those who shouted loudest, but those who lived consistently, often at cost. These are the witnesses. In D-Faith, they form the validation layer—drawing directly from the witness tradition that the Church has carried for centuries.

Testimony as Trust

In its ancient sense, *witness* was never passive. In Judaism, two witnesses confirmed truth. In Christianity, *martys* meant witness—proof by life. In Islam, the *Shahada* is both a declaration and an act of witnessing.

Testimony has always meant more than words. It meant: *I stake my life on this.*

In blockchain, proof-of-work means you've spent real energy validating something. In D-Faith, the analogue is spiritual cost: staying kind under pressure, forgiving when no one sees, and showing up when it would be easier to walk away.

Reputation isn't claimed. It's earned—block by block, through small acts that hold their shape under the slow audit of time.

From Metrics to Meaning

In a decentralised spiritual system, reputation becomes a shared record—an echo of the way the Church has long recognised saints, elders, and faithful members by the testimony of their lives—not performance, but consistency; not applause, but integrity.

Imagine:

— A ledger of moral actions, logged not to receive praise but to preserve memory.

— Peer-affirmed trust, where character is vouched for through lived witness.

— Zero-knowledge tools that verify presence without exposure—like the quiet glow of a candle seen through a veil.

For example, a D-Faith node might use zero-knowledge proof to confirm that a member has kept a private covenant—such as visiting the sick weekly for a year—without revealing who was visited or what was said. Two fellow members cryptographically co-sign the proof, which is time-stamped on the shared ledger. The act remains unseen, but the trust is real, verifiable, and anchored in community memory.

As both Epictetus and Marcus Aurelius wrote, virtue is seen in what we do when no one watches. In the same spirit, Jesus taught that when you give, let it be in secret—away from applause or credit[1].

Integrity and Its Risks

Every system carries temptations—ego, burnout, surveillance. That's why the witness layer must remain *sacred, but light:*

— No spiritual leaderboard.

— No martyrdom-for-status.

— No gatekeepers with hidden keys.

Decay over time prevents power from calcifying. Private proofs prevent exposure. Trust grows not by title, but by staying.

Incarnate, Not Abstract

For Bonhoeffer, the truest witness of faith was a life lived with integrity, not force or display.

In a world drowning in noise, the deepest proof is simple: a life aligned. The truth that persuades is not shouted, but lived. That's the witness layer. It stands alongside the Church's enduring witness as another way to recognise lives aligned with love and truth—that's D-Faith's proof-of-work.

---

1. *"When you give to the needy, do not let your left hand know what your right hand is doing, so that your giving may be in secret. Then your Father, who sees what is done in secret, will reward you."* (Matthew 6:3–4, NIV)

It's the kind of living that makes others wonder—gradually, with a curiosity they can't explain—if there might be more to trust and truth than they thought.

A changed, aligned, offered life—

That's the real proof-of-work.

And sometimes the truest proof-of-work is simply staying faithful when no one is watching. Whether in the quiet perseverance of a parish elder or the hidden constancy of a D-Faith participant, the same Spirit sustains the work.

Q: *If false virtue can't be fully prevented, is there value in third-party witnessing—and how could that actually work in a decentralised faith system?*

A: If someone writes a message into a decentralised faith ledger—a vow, a confession, a line from scripture—does it matter whether anyone else sees it? Can another person's awareness add meaning to what was recorded?

There's no guarantee that being seen will make a message more sincere. When someone else encounters what you've written—not in passing, but with attention—it moves the entry from private intent to shared memory. It doesn't confirm the truth of what you wrote, but—much like the role of a witness in the Church—it creates a reference point outside yourself. A tether. Something that remains visible, traceable, and a little harder to walk away from.

Some protocols may make this visible: a public ledger that others can explore, a logbook where responses unfold across time, or an attestation that records, "I saw this." These gestures don't judge. They don't endorse. But they do mark that something passed between people. That a message wasn't left to disappear. This kind of witnessing becomes part of the moral fabric—not by enforcing belief, but by anchoring memory—just as shared testimony and public confession have long strengthened the Church's life together.

Over time, a pattern can emerge—of those who write and return, and those who read and quietly witness. It's not a test. It's a structure. A network of expression and reception that adds weight to the messages it holds.

In this way, digital witnessing in D-Faith can sit alongside the embodied witness of gathered worship, each reinforcing the other in sustaining truth and memory.

For a deeper exploration, read "The Value in Witnessing" in the Bonus Materials.

Chapter 19

Open-Source Revelation

What if the sacred didn't come from above—but from among?

Core Problem or Tension: Religious truth has often been controlled, curated—and closed. Revelation was something dispensed from on high—interpreted by the few, enforced on the many. This centralised model of truth has alienated modern seekers who crave participation, not passive consumption.

What This Chapter Offers: A reimagining of revelation as an open-source phenomenon—ongoing, participatory, and distributed. Drawing from the ethos of collaborative software, this chapter proposes a living, editable, and community-vetted model of spiritual insight that aligns with decentralised faith.

Why It Matters Now: In a time when institutional authority is crumbling and spiritual hunger is rising, people are seeking fresh ways to access the sacred. This chapter offers an architecture of openness—where truth is shared, iterated, and tested in community, not dictated through hierarchy.

"The kingdom of God is within you."

—Luke 17:21

For most of history, revelation came from the top down—Moses with tablets, Muhammad in a cave, Joseph Smith with plates. In a preliterate

world, centralised authority made sense. But over time, insight hardened into dogma. As Karen Armstrong observed in *The Battle for God,* the further revelation travels from its source, the more it solidifies into control.

In a digital age—decentralised, networked, and suspicious of gatekeeping—truth may need a new shape.

Revelation as Participation

Revelation can be seen as a living process—gathered and refined over time, like a version-controlled document. Rooted in the wisdom of prophets and tradition, it continues to grow as communities reflect, contribute, and respond together.

What is sacred isn't only what was once received; it's also how that truth continues to be faithfully revisited and applied, in continuity with the traditions that have carried it.

Imagine:

— **A Sacred Wiki**, where spiritual insight is curated collaboratively, each edit signed and preserved in its lineage.

— **Revelation DAOs**, stewarding story and song like open-source scripture—seasonal psalms, shared prayers, annotated parables.

— **Proof-of-Insight Protocols**, where contributions are valued not by likes or those who shout loudest, but by long-term alignment, presence, and the fruit they bear over months or years.

This isn't chaos. It's *covenantal pluralism*—diverse voices orbiting shared values.

It also echoes history. Rabbinic scholars filled margins with debate. Monastics copied manuscripts, adding their own notes in the corners. Sufi mystics sang truths into memory. Indigenous elders carried wisdom in stories rather than statutes.

The sacred was always shared—often through the Church's stewardship and other faith traditions' care—it just wasn't always digital.

Mystery and Guardrails

But not everything sacred can, or should be explained. Many truths come wrapped in silence. D-Faith must resist the temptation to tokenise every insight or reduce reverence to metadata.

As much as we open-source theology, we must leave plenty of room for wonder.

That means building with guardrails:

— **Reputation** earned by practice, not profile.

— **Consensus** required for major changes.

— **Immutable logs** that preserve the entire history of ideas—so nothing is erased, only added to.

A parallel already exists in the digital commons. Wikipedia allows almost anyone to edit, but certain "protected pages" can only be changed after community agreement. These safeguards prevent vandalism without freezing the page forever. Likewise, in D-Faith, the most foundational insights could be open to discussion, yet require a clear threshold of shared trust before revision—protecting the root while letting new branches grow.

This isn't just about data integrity. It's about moral integrity. When someone returns to a passage years later, they should see not just the current words, but the journey—how interpretations shifted, where dissent sharpened the truth, and where humility said, "*We don't yet know.*"

Sacred knowledge will endure because of resonance. People return to what moves them. Not always immediately—but deeply, eventually.

Truth still speaks. Sometimes through code. Always through conscience.

In this unfolding process, sacred insight doesn't drift further from us—it draws closer.

The Kingdom isn't waiting at the edge of doctrine or behind institutional walls. It lives wherever wisdom is tended, shared, and made flesh—within and among us, version by version.

In this way, a decentralised approach can become another vineyard in which the same truth the Church has long proclaimed continues to grow—rooted in the same soil, branching into new spaces.

Q: *WHERE WOULD ALL THE SPIRITUAL ARTIFACTS—THE ORIGINAL TEXTS, SACRED FORKS, COMMENTARIES—ACTUALLY LIVE IN A SYSTEM LIKE D-FAITH? AND HOW WOULD A SEEKER FIND OR FOLLOW THEM?*

A: In traditional religion, sacred wisdom is stored in scrolls and scriptures, safeguarded in temples, churches, monasteries, and libraries. In D-Faith, that memory would live differently—not in a central vault, but across a network of references. Each points. Each preserves.

A blockchain can't carry the full weight of a thousand pages, but it can hold the fingerprint of a truth. The foundational document—the Genesis Protocol—might live on a distributed file system like IPFS. So would its forks, revisions, and annotations. The blockchain itself would store the cryptographic record: not the content, but proof of its authenticity and its moment in time.

You wouldn't need permission or status—just genuine curiosity. The trail's there: open, visible, and maybe a bit winding. One link leads to another. Meaning meanders, as it should, through a living faith.

Some seekers might follow curated paths—annotated trails of resonance, peer-vouched nodes, or collections of sacred insight shaped by community attention over time.

What emerges isn't a fixed canon, but a living archive—held in shared responsibility, and able to sit alongside the fixed canon and sacred tradition that the Church continues to preserve.

Best of all, truth lives where no one can erase it, and in this design, the enduring witness of the Church and the distributed memory of D-Faith can reinforce one another—each protecting the truth in its own way.

For a deeper exploration, read "Where The Artifacts Live" in the Bonus Materials.

Chapter 20

Forking With Integrity—

When Conviction and Conscience Diverge

Core Problem or Tension: In a decentralised faith system, spiritual divergence is not only possible—it's anticipated. But if every difference of conscience results in a split, what keeps the community whole? What stops fragmentation from becoming erosion?

What This Chapter Offers: A deeper exploration of "forking" as a sacred responsibility within D-Faith. It reframes divergence as an opportunity when anchored in integrity. As the moral-architectural blueprint for responsible divergence, **i**t's about *how* to leave well when conscience demands it. Importantly, it also explores what Bitcoin teaches us about stability at scale.

Why It Matters Now: As consensus culture gives way to individualised truth, many institutions break under the strain. Traditional religions splinter. Political movements radicalise. In D-Faith, we don't just need the tools to agree—we need the wisdom to part ways well.

"The enthusiasts of liberty thought they were leaving it unlimited, when they were only leaving it undefined. They thought they were leaving it undefined, when they were really leaving it undefended."

— G.K. Chesterton

Every enduring tradition reaches a crossroads: to reform, fracture, or fossilise. D-Faith introduces another path—*to fork with integrity*: a way to diverge when conscience calls, without breaking the sacred thread that binds.

Divergence with Reverence

Faith has always adapted, sometimes through division. Christianity's history includes the East–West Schism and the Protestant Reformation—moments of pain and renewal that still sit within God's ongoing work through His Church. Islam divided into Sunni and Shia, and Buddhism into Theravāda and Mahāyāna. These were not just doctrinal clashes but collisions of conscience, power, and identity.

The real loss wasn't disagreement—it was when disagreement led to exile.

In D-Faith, divergence is expected—and when grounded in shared covenant, it can be an act of fidelity, not rebellion.

Integrity begins with posture. To fork well is to:

— Honour your roots, even as you grow elsewhere.

— Explain your reasoning, not just pronounce it.

— Invite response, diffuse retaliation.

— Carry your story, rather than erase it.

The process may need to be methodical, but the resulting benefits are very human. Forking isn't just a tech function—it's a sacred tension between continuity and conscience. It asks what you believe, why you must walk differently, and whether you can still walk with love.

In D-Faith, disagreement doesn't threaten unity; it tests it. Different nodes might live the covenant in distinct ways—some contemplative, others activist; some minimalist, others mystical. This isn't relativism—it's **covenantal pluralism**. What binds is not sameness, but sincerity.

When Divergence Feels Like Exile

We must be honest: not every fork will feel mutually beneficial. Some may dominate public discourse or cultural power, leaving others displaced. Consider modern debates around marriage or identity—where once-majority views now carry social risk. For some, this shift feels like renewal. For others, it feels like exile.

D-Faith can't erase this grief. But it can record it with dignity.

Every fork—whether generative or painful—is documented in the Sacred Record:

— What changed?

— What was grieved?

— What still remains in honour.

This practice works much like *Git's commit history* in open-source software: even when a project branches, the record of why and how it diverged is preserved forever. Memory becomes the antidote to erasure. Divergence becomes part of continuity.

Discernment, Not Drama

D-Faith may avoid gatekeeping—but it still requires discernment. Forks aren't immune to ego, opportunism, or spiritual manipulation. That's why transparency matters more than control.

Each fork must reference its origins. Its witnesses. Its intention.

As in blockchain or open-source software, some forks will thrive; others will fade—not by censorship but by exposure. In time, people will follow the paths they trust—not necessarily the most powerful, but the most fruitful.

Three Illustrative Forks

— **Ethical Minimalists** distill the covenant into five clear principles—seeking simplicity, not rebellion.

— **Communalists** integrate economics and spirituality by practising resource-sharing and collective labour.

— **AI Mystics** explore revelation through sacred prompting and artificial intelligence.

These are illustrations only. Each is distinct, yet all honour the covenant, act transparently, and invite honest engagement.

Toward Fertile Fracture

We've been taught to fear splits as threats. But sometimes, fracture fertilises.

Jesus brought the fulfilment of God's covenant within Judaism. The Buddha stepped beyond Vedic tradition. Martin Luther, Dorothy Day, and Martin Luther King Jr. worked for renewal within the faith they loved, seeking reform rather than rejection. They walked away not in anger but in faithfulness—to carry forward what others had forgotten.

To fork with reverence is to say, *This matters enough to change for—but not to discard.*

Chesterton's Warning

Chesterton warned that undefined liberty becomes undefended liberty. The same is true in faith. When traditions fear divergence, they risk stagnation. But when they allow every fork to become law, they risk erosion.

D-Faith defends sacredness not through gatekeeping but through *memory, conscience, and voluntary trust.* No voice rules, but every voice is recorded.

Forks, when guided by prayer, humility, and conscience, can be part of how God preserves and renews His Church and other faith communities.

Let them come—not to scatter us, but to multiply what we dare to call holy.

Postscript: What Bitcoin Teaches About Stability at Scale

"As the network grows, it becomes more conservative."
— Bitcoin Core Advocate

This insight from cryptocurrency isn't just about economics. It's about social inertia, accumulated trust, and the cost of walking away from something proven.

In open-source technology, forking is a design feature: you can copy the codebase, take it elsewhere, and build something new. In blockchain, this has led to famous splits—like Bitcoin vs. Bitcoin Cash—each representing a different philosophy.

But over time, the larger the network, the more conservative it becomes.

When Bitcoin forked in 2017, the result was two chains:

— **Bitcoin (BTC)** kept the original rules—prioritising security, decentralisation, and deliberate evolution.

— **Bitcoin Cash (BCH)** prioritised faster transactions and bigger block sizes.

Initially, both were viable. Both claimed fidelity to Satoshi's vision. But years later, only one carried the full weight of history. BTC continued to attract users, developers, and capital. BCH still exists, but never regained the cultural gravity of the original.

Why? Because once a network has enough participants, memory, and momentum, a fork is no longer just a technical change—it's a moral and relational fracture. Leaving isn't "wrong," but it's costly unless there's no alternative.

This is *path dependence*: the idea that past choices shape present possibilities. Each step down a path:

— Builds **infrastructure** (literal or symbolic)

— Creates **expectations** and **routines**

— Accumulates **investments** (emotional, social, economic)

In faith, the same dynamic holds. If a community has lived under one covenant for decades—shaping rituals, songs, and testimony—then even a small deviation can feel like a betrayal. Not because the new path is unworthy, but because the old one has roots.

From Bitcoin to D-Faith

In the early days of a D-Faith protocol, forking may be frequent. Communities will:

— Test new Genesis Documents

— Remix liturgies and rituals

— Adjust primitives like what counts as witness, covenant, or sacred service

This is natural and even good—the early network is experimental, light to lift, and lineage is thin.

But as one fork matures, *spiritual gravity* sets in. Testimony accumulates. Disputes and reconciliations are logged. Children inherit not just practices but memory. Forking becomes possible but weighty.

Fork Resistance in Practice

Fork resistance is the growing reluctance to split as a network gains size and value. It emerges through:

1. **Ritual Legitimacy** – Practices lived and witnessed develop reverent inertia.

2. **Covenantal Memory** – A shared archive of belief, dispute, and reconciliation forms.

3. **Intergenerational Transmission** – Traditions become embedded in identity.

4. **Spiritual & Social Capital** – Contribution becomes moral currency; leaving spends it.

5. **Coordination Cost & Network Inertia** – Large, distributed networks resist disruption—not by forbidding dissent, but by making change consequential.

This produces *dynamic conservatism*: stability earned, not enforced. D-Faith doesn't forbid forks—it simply makes the careless ones, or those driven by an ideologically driven minority, expensive.

The longer a lineage endures, the more leaving it means detaching from the memory, trust, and life you helped build. In this way, D-Faith's approach to forking can echo the Church's own call to unity in essentials, liberty in non-essentials, and charity in all things—honouring conscience while protecting the bonds of peace.

In Chapter Six, we considered how institutional drift has been playing out in the 21st century. At the end of this chapter, it's worth asking ourselves how forces like path dependence and resistance to forking might shape a decentralised faith community—especially one where decisions aren't dictated from above, but emerge through participatory consensus?

Even in the face of activism or political pressure, such a system would allow the community to support its fork by showing up and voting through presence.

Q: *What might it feel like to experience a fork in D-Faith?*

A: It may begin quietly—an update, a reflection, a shift in tone. You learn that a new path has emerged. Not a rupture with the Gospel or the core of the faith, but a realignment in emphasis, expression, or practice—a fork.

At first, it might feel disorienting. Something you thought was shared now bends in two directions. You may feel curious, unsettled, affirmed, or deeply moved. It's okay to feel all of it.

You are not required to take sides. You can remain precisely where you are. The original fork continues. Your presence still matters. Your record remains whole.

Some will explore the new branch, others will stay rooted, and many will pause to discern. There is no punishment for staying, no guilt for leaving, and no erasure either way.

Through it all, the system bears witness—not to division but to devotion shaped differently. It holds space for the truth that even when paths diverge in expression, each can still be faithful to the same Lord and sacred calling.

For those who choose to remain?

In a well-designed spiritual or ideological fork, the original resources and infrastructure should remain accessible to both sides, unless deliberately severed.

This mirrors how forks work in open-source software or blockchains: the **original chain doesn't disappear**, and those who fork can still read, reference, or even sync with the earlier version. A healthy fork doesn't erase the past—it builds on it, choosing a different future while remaining connected to the same foundation.

In D-Faith terms, this means:

— **Scripture, teachings, community contributions, and sacred records** from before the fork are still visible and accessible, unless a new community decides to hide or overwrite them (which would violate transparency).

— **Shared tooling or rituals** (e.g., smart covenant formats, pseudonym graphs, consensus tools) can still be used, though they may be modified downstream.

— **Participants retain agency**: some may straddle both traditions, acting as bridges or memory-keepers between the forked paths.

So yes—continuity is preserved, but direction may diverge. That's what makes it a fork, not a rupture. In this way, D-Faith forks can reflect the Church's own history of renewal movements and local adaptations—different branches, still drawing from the same root.

For a deeper exploration, read "What a Fork Might Feel Like in D-Faith" in the Bonus Materials.

Chapter 21

Sacred Protocols

— Not New Religions

Core Problem or Tension: Every spiritual movement faces the risk of becoming what it once resisted. Innovation turns into orthodoxy. Revelation becomes ritual. The sacred, once fluid and alive, hardens into an institution. D-Faith must confront this tendency not as an anomaly, but as a design challenge.

What This Chapter Offers: A vision of spiritual life built not on institutions, but on *sacred protocols*—practices and principles that evolve through community, conscience, and participation. It draws from open-source systems and covenantal traditions to propose a way of structuring faith that resists rigidity without losing reverence.

Why It Matters Now: In an era where people seek meaning without control, ritual without rigidity, and truth without tyranny, this chapter offers a pathway to practice and belonging that avoids the traps of empire thinking. It explains how to protect the sacred not through power, but through design.

"Institutions try to preserve the problem to which they are the solution."

— Stewart Brand

Every movement faces a moment when inspiration risks hardening into control. Religions, like software, suffer *version lock*—not from failure to innovate, but from the dominance of their earliest innovations. What began as a flame, in time, becomes ash.

Jesus overturned tables to restore worship to its rightful focus; centuries later, human ambition sometimes used his name in conquest—forgetting the servant-leadership he modelled. The Buddha offered liberation; over time, the dharma calcified into hierarchy. Even secular visions weren't immune: the Enlightenment's pursuit of reason hardened into elite institutions. Early internet idealism has been swallowed by surveillance capitalism.

D-Faith must not reject the structures God has used to preserve faith, but supplement them with a new kind—alive, adaptive, and protective without possession. Not a new religion, but sacred protocols that can renew and reinforce the life of the Church.

What Is a Sacred Protocol?

A protocol is how communities align without control—consensual frameworks for discernment, practice, and change. In the technical world, TCP/IP lets every internet-connected device "speak" without a central authority. Ethereum's EIP (Ethereum Improvement Proposal) process allows anyone to suggest changes, but nothing is adopted without visible, community-wide agreement.

Sacred protocols work the same way—spiritual code that is flexible, revisable, and grounded in shared values. They function like GitHub repositories, open to contributions, versioned transparently, and forkable when needed.

Examples:

Ethical Commitment Protocol: Members sign a covenantal statement, such as "*truth over popularity*," visible on a ledger and periodically renewed.

Ritual Proposal Protocol: A participant suggests a communal practice; if the group affirms it, it becomes part of the node's shared rhythm.

— *Dispute Navigation Protocol:* Disagreements handled through peer circles, witnesses, and rest periods—not edicts. Only the process is recorded, not the conflict.

These aren't abstractions. They are living forms of memory, stored in decentralised formats (GitHub, IPFS, Arweave), sitting at the edge of trust and visibility.

Not a System, an Ecosystem

D-Faith isn't a denomination—it's a network of spiritually aligned communities, each free to remain in fellowship with the wider Church while living out the Gospel in locally authentic ways. Protocols are the pollinators. One community's dispute process might inspire another's, just as one tree's blossoms feed a whole habitat. Energy flows through *reputation*, not bureaucratic authority.

A sacred protocol often emerges from a felt need—renewal, tension, or transition—and becomes a shared reference point for onboarding, moments of conflict, or when a community re-commits.

To uphold one is to make a vow:

— I act with integrity, because I believe it is holy.

— I fork if needed, but never from ego.

— I join rituals that nourish, not dominate.

— I build memory to forget less and forgive more.

This isn't solely infrastructure for belief—it's also design for continuity. Like the Hippocratic Oath or Creative Commons, its strength is in voluntary alignment.

Toward the Living Covenant

At the heart is covenant—not fixed, but living. Written in action. Re-committed by choice. Remembered in the chain.

Brand warned that institutions tend to preserve the problems they were built to solve. Sacred protocols subvert that fate. They are not de-

signed to last forever—they are designed to evolve, with a trail honest enough for others to begin again.

D-Faith's deepest promise?

That truth need not calcify.

That reverence can survive decentralisation.

That the sacred may breathe better when no one owns it—and when the code is written so that, unlike institutions, it never has to defend itself by keeping the problem alive. In this way, sacred protocols become tools of reformation in the truest sense—helping the Body of Christ stay supple, truthful, and united in its mission, even as it adapts to new challenges.

Q: *What might God think of Decentralised Faith?*

A: If D-Faith is more than just a novel experiment in spiritual structure, we must ask—not presume—what might God think of this project? Not in theory, but how a child might glance at a parent after doing something bold. Is this an act of faithful evolution—or misdirected ambition?

Scripture offers clues. Again and again, God's attention seems less fixed on form and more on fruit—less on structure and more on mercy. *"I desire mercy, not sacrifice,"* says Hosea. Micah distills it further: *act justly, love mercy, walk humbly.* Jesus directs His sharpest rebukes not at outsiders but at insiders—those who burden others with rules while shutting the door of the Kingdom in their faces. He wasn't angered by change but by control disguised as holiness.

Whatever it may be, this project must not fall into that trap. If D-Faith becomes another mechanism for exclusion, pride, or performance, then it risks becoming Babel rebranded—unity without humility, progress without purpose. But if it opens up shared responsibility, reduces the distance between soul and Source, and creates space for belonging, then perhaps it reflects something God has long hoped His people might attempt—in harmony with the mission He has entrusted to His Church through every age.

"You are a royal priesthood," Peter wrote—not a congregation beneath a pulpit, but a distributed holiness, lived through ordinary lives. Our tools may be new, but the heart must remain ancient.

We're not here to build a tower apart from Him. We're here to set a table where the Body of Christ, in all its diversity, can gather and grow. And if what grows from this is love, joy, patience, and peace, then perhaps God not only permits it. Perhaps He delights in it.▯

For a deeper exploration, *read "Divine Sanction or Divine Adaptation?" in the Bonus Materials.*

Q: *WITHOUT OFFICIAL ID HOW DO YOU KNOW I'M ME?*

A: Because over time, we leave more than a name. We leave patterns, like how we ask questions, show up, and respond when no one's watching.

A soulful pseudonym isn't just a chosen name; it's a *continuity signal* that allows you to grow without breaking the thread of trust.

And when someone uses a mask to deceive, it doesn't stay hidden forever.

The community begins to sense it: promises made but never lived, words repeated without substance, gestures that gather goodwill but never return it.

The ledger keeps record, but only of what's written.

It keeps a trail of what we say.

What we've done, and what we've truly lived.

That's why trust in D-Faith isn't built from data alone. It's built from discernment.

Over time, those who walk with integrity begin to shine.

And those who don't? The pattern speaks for itself.

Because in a shared memory system, truth has company. And light, though quiet, keeps seeking.

For a deeper exploration, *read "How do you know I'm me?" in the Bonus Materials.*

Q: *WHAT'S TO STOP SOMEONE FROM USING A PSEUDONYM TO LIE, POSTURE, OR DECEIVE?*

A: This is a real risk—and pretending otherwise would be naive.

Pseudonymity, without anchoring, becomes cosplay (costume play), a spiritual mask. You can craft the perfect version of yourself—post beautiful reflections, join rituals, even mentor others—without ever showing who you truly are. And if no one can see the gaps between what you say and how you live, trust collapses. It's not just hollow. It's dangerous.

That's why D-Faith doesn't stop at pseudonymity. It *starts* there. The system isn't built on performative profiles but on tethered presence.

Every soulful pseudonym is meant to be tethered to a *small, stable circle* of others who can vouch for your consistency, not through surveillance, but through genuine relationship. Not everyone sees everything. But someone who walks with you does. And over time, *your reputation isn't just what you say—it's what others see, remember, and* privately *affirm.* This isn't about panopticon-style transparency. It's about trust that comes from being known over time.

A pseudonym without tethering is just another brand. But a pseudonym anchored in small, discerning circles—that's where depth lives.

If you're the only one writing your story, there's no contradiction, or growth. But when your voice is part of a thread woven with others—seen, remembered, *witnessed*—the story starts gaining weight.

And yes, D-Faith is digital, but it isn't *disembodied.* The goal isn't to replace embodied fellowship or the life of the Church. It's to decentralise spiritual memory so it can complement the witness of the Church across generations. It's to decentralise *spiritual memory*—to ensure that wisdom, ritual, and presence can live and move across time and place, not die with institutions.

So, how do we prevent deceit? We rely on people. Small circles. Long arcs. Mutual memory. That's where the soul of D-Faith lives—not in code alone, but in the company it keeps.

For other safeguards, including *cryptographic identity* tools, go to the chapter "*Beyond Evangelism...*"

Chapter 22

The Remnant and the Revival

Where the future begins again—with those who never stopped remembering.

Core Problem or Tension: When dominant systems decay or collapse, hope can feel impossible. Yet history shows that renewal often begins not at the center, but at the edges—with those who remember.

What This Chapter Offers: An exploration of "the remnant" in spiritual, cultural, and technological terms. It highlights those who preserve wisdom through decline and become seeds of future revival—from Amish farmers to digital monks.

Why It Matters Now: As institutions fail and myths crumble, the future belongs to those who can remember what mattered—and live it faithfully in small, resilient ways.

> *"Hope is not the conviction that something will turn out well, but the certainty that something is worth doing, no matter how it turns out."*
>
> — Vaclav Havel

Throughout history, when institutions collapse or lose moral clarity, a remnant remains. Not always loud or visible, but faithful. They hold what matters when others move on. This chapter is about them—those who remember, and through remembering, help renew.

In the early 6th century, Benedict of Nursia withdrew from a disintegrating Roman world. From his quiet retreat came a rhythm of life—work, prayer, hospitality—that would outlast the empire. The Quakers, centuries later, designed leaderless gatherings based on silence and consensus. Others—like the Anabaptists or early Methodists—formed small, local communities with shared spiritual practice and mutual accountability.

These weren't movements for their own sake. They were responses to dislocation, each rooted in spiritual rhythm rather than institutional ambition.

The same impulse is alive today. It's found in those who shape their lives intentionally—in family homes, co-living groups, farms, studios, servers. Not rejecting the world, but choosing how to live within it.

The Digital Remnant

Some of today's remnant are builders—writing open-source code or creating decentralised tools for shared decision-making. Others keep a candlelit table or a Sabbath phone basket. They may not call it spiritual, but they are attending to the same questions:

— What forms help meaning take root?

— What is worth preserving, repeating, or passing on?

The Amish offer a useful case. Often caricatured, they're not anti-technology—they critically evaluate it. Will this tool serve the community, or erode it? Phones are allowed in barns, but not kitchens. Decisions are made locally, not nationally. Their discernment is quiet, values-led, and collective. It works not because it scales, but because it's clear and consistent.

A similar discernment is appearing in digital communities. On the decentralised social platform Mastodon, each "instance" sets its own norms and chooses which others to connect with—or block—based on shared values. Secure Scuttlebutt, a peer-to-peer social protocol, lets communities communicate and coordinate even offline, ensuring resilience where global networks can't be trusted. In both cases, the

test isn't technical novelty, but whether the tool deepens trust and strengthens the culture it serves.

D-Faith's remnant will likely use the same principle—choosing protocols, rituals, and tools not because they are fashionable, but because they are worth carrying forward.

Similar patterns are emerging in urban and digital settings. Some groups share meals and prayers in small houses. Others design digital spaces for sacred conversation or mutual care. These aren't nostalgic reenactments—they are live, local responses to a changing world. They remember that meaning requires form, and form requires rhythm.

The biblical idea of the "remnant" speaks directly to this. From Israel's prophets to the house churches of the New Testament, the remnant has always been God's instrument for carrying His covenant through times of trial. What they preserved was not just culture, but God's own promises. Isaiah used the term 'remnant' to describe a faithful few who endured when others turned away. The Apostle Paul saw it as continuity—threads held through history. Not elite. Not idealised. But committed.

Historian Arnold Toynbee called such groups "creative minorities"—small communities that preserve what matters through cultural disruption. Their power lies not in numbers but in coherence. Imperfect, but with clear direction.

In our time, the remnant may include digital builders, slow readers, co-housing neighbours, or anyone asking: How should we live now?

Disconnection also plays a role. As Ivan Illich once wrote, the most radical move is not confrontation, but withdrawal—the refusal to be shaped entirely by systems that distort. Even Jesus, we're told, withdrew to lonely places to pray. Silence was not absence—it was part of the work.

What matters isn't whether these lives are noticed, but whether they are faithful. They are not waiting to be rescued or platformed. They're planting something lasting. They carry questions that don't age:

— *What do I owe others?*

— *What is worth repeating?*

— *How do we build something we'd trust our children to inherit?*

These are not nostalgic questions. They are seeds. Revival rarely begins at the centre. They aren't certain of outcomes. They aren't promised success.

Seeds of a New Reformation

We build anyway—homes, habits, lines of code, shared meals. Not because we know it will work, but because we believe it's worth doing.

As Vaclav Havel reminded us, hope is not the guarantee of success—it's the conviction that some things are worth doing, even if the harvest comes long after we are gone. The remnant lives by that conviction, planting anyway, not driven solely by optimism, but unrelenting fidelity.

Revival takes root in remembering—when those few who still carry the flame choose to build again, not as it was, but in renewed faithfulness to God's heart and purposes, as they were meant to be.

Chapter 23

The "Greater Than" Principle

Core Problem or Tension: We live in an age of collapse—in (truthful) shared stories, and common cause. People aren't just disconnected from one another, but from purpose itself. At the heart of our disorientation lies a forgotten truth: the human soul needs something to serve that is greater than itself.

What This Chapter Offers: The "Greater Than" Principle—the idea that deep meaning, personal integrity, and communal cohesion only emerge when individuals orient themselves toward a transcendent reference point. Drawing from psychology, theology and technology, it proposes that fulfillment comes not through self-actualization, but self-transcendence.

Why It Matters Now: Flooded with choices but deprived of direction, the self has become the center of the moral universe. The rise in anxiety, division, and spiritual numbness signals a loss of orientation. Reclaiming transcendence may anchor life in purpose beyond personal success.

"For success, like happiness, cannot be pursued; it must ensue... as the unintended side effect of one's personal dedication to a cause greater than oneself."

— Viktor E. Frankl

We live in a time marked by collapse—not just of institutions but of shared stories and moral orientation. Knowledge is abundant; compass points are not. What's missing isn't intellect. It's transcendence.

As Frankl learned in the aftermath of the Holocaust, meaning does not appear through direct pursuit. It emerges when life is oriented toward something greater than the self. Yet today, many arrange their lives around metrics, identity, or distraction rather than God, covenant, or the common good. The result is fragmentation—systems built on the self cannot bear their own weight.

The *Greater Than* Principle insists that fulfillment and stability arise only when we are aligned with something that will outlast us. Abraham Maslow's late work placed self-transcendence above self-actualisation; in spiritual terms, it means asking not only *how* to restore the sacred, but *why* it is worth serving at all. Transcendence is not only vertical; it is connective—binding us to one another in shared purpose.

The best systems—spiritual, social, or technological—point beyond the self. Twelve-step recovery begins with surrender to a Higher Power. Good parenting de-centres the adult in favour of the child. The Amish live by *Ordnung*—a moral code that resists efficiency for the sake of endurance, setting limits freely embraced rather than externally imposed.

In D-Faith, the same impulse can be seen in miniature:

—*The Shared Table Node*: a group that meets weekly for a simple meal, each bringing a dish and a brief reflection. Attendance isn't tracked, but every shared evening is logged in the Sacred Record as a "hospitality block." The point isn't credit—it's continuity. Over time, the record becomes a testimony of care that spans years.

—*The Repair Chain*: a network of craftworkers, farmers, and coders who pledge a set number of hours each month to repairing tools, clothing, or code for others in the community. The repairs are logged on-chain, not to show off, but so that future members inherit a lineage of service—evidence that the covenant was lived, not just spoken.

These are small acts, but they are deliberately tethered to something *greater than the participants themselves*. They don't measure success by how much attention they get, but by the integrity of what they pass on.

D-Faith is designed in the same spirit as the Church at its best: to reignite faith in Christianity and restore moral orientation in decentralised form, complementing and strengthening the witness of existing congregations rather than replacing them. Here, protocols are not just technical but covenantal. Consensus encodes memory. Blockchains become testaments. *Greater Than* becomes moral architecture: your commitments are witnessed, your service is remembered, and your life is oriented toward what you will never fully own.

Awe is part of this design. Dacher Keltner's research shows awe reduces ego and fosters generosity; sacred traditions call it the beginning of wisdom. In D-Faith, awe is built into the structure—not as spectacle, but as a rhythm that draws us out of ourselves and back into reverence.

To live by the *Greater Than* Principle is far beyond questions of submission—it is natural alignment. It means shaping our days around what will endure, orienting our work toward the communal, and anchoring ourselves in the sacred. As Rabbi Jonathan Sacks said, "The greatest single antidote to violence is a sense of shared meaning."

So the question returns to each of us:

What is so precious you would guard it at great cost?

What truth stands higher than your own success?

What future is worth giving yourself to?

Frankl's answer was clear—and it remains a challenge to us today. Meaning is never the goal. It is a by-product of what happens when you live for something *greater than yourself*.

"The Record of Ruth"

A short story of a believer in transition

Setting: Suburban England, present day

Characters:

— **Ruth**, late 30s, raised Anglican, recently re-engaging with her faith

— **Mark**, her vicar, kind, sincere, stretched thin

"Ecclesia", an anonymous online fellowship of believers using a decentralised faith protocol

Part I: Unsettled

Ruth sat at the back of St. Anne's, as she had done most Sundays since Christmas. The hymns were familiar, and the prayers were soothing. Morning light bathed the stained glass in soft color.

But something felt missing — like eating food that looked nourishing but left her empty.

The sermons were kind, but cautious. The community was warm, but not intimate. And more than once, she'd wondered:

"Is this the real faith... or just a copy of a copy?"

She didn't doubt God. She questioned the institution — or at least its ability to speak to her heart, to her time.

Part II: Whispering Code

One evening, scrolling through a theology forum, she saw a strange invitation:

"Join a Church no one can own. Where every soul writes their own scroll. Where Scripture lives forever — and no pastor can erase your voice."

It led to something called *Ecclesia* — not a new denomination, but a protocol.

She almost closed the tab. But curiosity... and a flicker of longing... held her hand.

Part III: Invisible Gathering

She created a faith identity — just "Ruth" — no surname, no bio. She joined a "Fellowship of the Cloud of Witnesses," a digital chapel of believers who studied scripture, shared reflections, and immutably logged their spiritual milestones.

Here's what she did in her first month:

Forked the Gospel of John, adding her own notes in the margins

Read a prayer left by a Syrian woman who had fled persecution

Attended a virtual communion circle led by a farmer in a neighboring region

Logged her confirmation from 1999 into the ledger — not for others, but to remember who she was

It was strange. It was quiet. It felt more tangible and authentic than anything she'd known since childhood.

Part IV: Confession

One night, after a fight with her brother, she wrote a prayer—not a polished one, but raw, angry, and grieving. She encrypted it and recorded it on the chain.

And something happened.

She didn't just feel heard by God. She felt held by time, by the community, by the quiet permanence of the record.

It was like placing grief in a vault lined with velvet. Or planting memory where no wind could blow it away.

Part V: Amplification

She didn't stop going to St. Anne's.

In fact, she began going more, but it was different now. She brought her reflections from *Ecclesia* into the Bible study. She spoke with Mark gently about transparency, scripture access, and shared leadership.

And over time, something opened.

She helped others in her church create "spiritual scrolls." Young people logged their baptisms. Elders preserved old teachings. Doubters left anonymous psalms.

What had been missing wasn't doctrine, or music, or ritual.

It was the sense that *faith belongs to everyone*.

That no one could edit your walk with God. No one could gate-keep your connection to God.

And now, they had found a way to hold that again. Together.

Epilogue:

Ruth logs in each morning and lights a virtual candle. It's never required. But it's always sincere and grounding.

A flame in a network of invisible hands. A chapel without walls. A Church that cannot fall.

PART III: IMAGINATION & IMPLEMENTATION

(Toward the Future)

“We shape our tools and thereafter our tools shape us.”

— Marshall McLuhan

Chapter 24

What Would It Feel Like?

— And Why Remain?

Core Problem or Tension: A decentralised faith system cannot succeed on technology alone. It must answer a deeper question: Without churches or clergy, can it meet the emotional, spiritual, and relational needs that have always drawn people to religion—and will they stay?

What This Chapter Offers: This chapter brings the abstract to life. It imagines what daily spiritual practice might look like in a decentralised faith system—how people might pray, gather, reflect, and contribute. It shows how meaning emerges not from structure, but from shared rhythm and remembered presence.

Why It Matters Now: In a world that moves fast and forgets easily, people are looking for something steady and sacred. This chapter argues that decentralised tools, if used with care, can offer more than function—they can help restore memory, deepen connection, and carry faith into daily life. Without this, D-Faith won't feel real enough to hold anyone.

"Play long-term games with long-term people."

— Naval Ravikant

In every generation, people seek not only beliefs but a way to live—something they can return to and rely on in times of joy and loss. Religion has often answered this longing through rhythm, ritual, and awe, so if a decentralised spiritual system is to matter, it must do the same. Protocols alone cannot sustain people. What will endure is meaning.

Throughout history, people have turned to faith because it meets their deepest longings:

To feel less alone in the universe when life seems random or crushing;

To make sense of suffering, giving pain a frame that doesn't destroy;

To find a moral compass—how to forgive, act justly, or live well;

To belong to something larger than themselves—not just a group, but a story, a lineage, a mission that carries identity beyond ambition.

Faith has also given us ways to feel clean again, to release the burden of guilt or regret. It has marked time with meaning, so that births, marriages, and deaths are not just events but sacred milestones. It has offered a language for awe when wonder overwhelms—at the stars, the ocean, the sight of new life. It has promised remembrance: that our lives will not simply vanish but will be held in memory. It has also suggested order, coherence, and a hunger for the holy that lies beyond transaction or utility.

Churches, mosques, temples, and synagogues have long met these needs—often beautifully, and at times imperfectly. The question now is whether a decentralised faith can help meet these needs effectively, with the same dignity, and gravity, and in ways that complement the life of the Church.

A Day in the Life

Imagine waking early. There is no bell tower or call to prayer, yet rhythm draws you back. You record a prayer or line of gratitude, a simple offering to God and time. It is yours, yet now it is remembered in a way that cannot be erased.

Later, you open a forked text maintained by a community you trust. Notes left by strangers carry weight: "*This verse saved me when my mother died.*" Their story becomes part of yours.

You gather with others, perhaps in a living room or a secure digital space. There is no ordained leader, only those who have earned trust through presence. Someone reads, another sings, another confesses doubt. It might not always be polished, but it will be real.

Elsewhere, someone is baptised. Her name is hidden, and her location is unclear, but her act of witness is permanent. It cost her something, and yet she still chose it.

You might contribute—translating a text, annotating a line, or lighting a digital candle with a one-line prayer. None of these alone may be grand gestures, but each becomes part of something larger than you.

Rhythm, Reverence, and Sacrifice

Rhythm keeps people tethered to faith—the daily, weekly, and seasonal patterns that become tradition. D-Faith doesn't need to invent new rituals; it can host those we already know, while letting communities fork and form new observances.

Reverence, too, emerges in the weight of permanence. A prayer written into a shared ledger feels different because it will not vanish. In a world built for forgetting, permanence itself becomes sacred.

And always, there is sacrifice. Faith has never come cheap. A pilgrim walking for days, a monk surrendering ambition, or today, someone logging into a system despite risk—all mark devotion. Even the simple act of pausing to record truth in D-Faith can be a form of offering.

Why Stay?

People won't stay for novelty. They will remain only if they sense that it matters—if their entries and rituals become part of a fabric larger than themselves. D-Faith can provide this by holding memory without

manipulation, preserving presence without demanding power, and offering participation without needing anyone's authorisation.

At its best, it becomes a place where someone responds, where prayers echo beyond the moment, and where the sacred is remembered—not replacing the role of Church and tradition, but adding a new layer of chain and covenant that can travel where institutions cannot. Their private life with God, far from being isolated, is accompanied, even if only through the possibility of being seen, remembered, and traced.

A New Book of Acts

Picture the early church and the earliest believers: small gatherings, handwritten letters, and lives shared in secret. They weren't safe or rewarded, but they believed in something that had to be recorded, passed on, preserved.

Now imagine those same people with access to a decentralised ledger—a gospel that could be forked but never burned, a psalm that could be stored uncensored for eternity.

D-Faith extends belief into a new layer—one that offers a bridge for those seeking a way back, carrying them toward the living memory that is still alive within their tradition, but may need renewed accessibility in a digital age. Naval Ravikant's counsel to *"play long-term games with long-term people"* is as true in faith as in life. In D-Faith, the "games" are covenants, rituals, and acts of service—pursued for endurance rather than short-term reward. The "people" are those who keep showing up—recording, remembering, and living what they profess—so that the chain of trust and reverence stretches far beyond any single life.

Q: *What does it really mean to "record presence" in a decentralised faith system? Why does it matter if no one sees it?*

A: In much of life, visibility is mistaken for value. If it's not liked, shared, or acknowledged, we're taught it didn't really happen. But that's not how memory, or conscience, or spirit work.

Recording presence isn't about seeking attention—it's about testifying to existence. It's a personal claim: *I was here. I chose. I believed. I acted.* Even if no one responds. Even if no one ever reads it. Placing that mark—especially into something enduring—can be a way of affirming truth to yourself and something beyond yourself.

It's not a transaction. It's a spiritual assertion that meaning exists whether or not it's seen.

The message doesn't have to be public to matter. It has to be real—because that's what D-Faith is built to preserve: not the spectacle of belief, but its substance—strengthening the living witness of Christianity by ensuring moments of faith are remembered and carried forward.

Q: *How do the physical gatherings of faith and the digital architecture of D-Faith actually work together?*

A: Faith has always been both personal and shared. You need conviction in your heart—and connection with those around you. A personal relationship with God gives direction; a collective rhythm with others gives it shape.

We grow through meet-ups, not downloads. Eye contact. Laughter. A quiet conversation after someone breaks down. These aren't just warm moments—they're the raw material of real community. The

physical side of faith is where trust is felt. The digital layer simply remembers it. It holds the words spoken, the vows made, the wisdom passed down—serving as a companion to the Church's wider story, helping consecrate the moment and ensure it endures for future believers.

And over time, those moments stack up. They become culture. They teach our children what matters. They remind us who we are.

This is how civilisations are built—not just through law or infrastructure, but through transcendence lived together. A pursuit held in common. Something sacred. When people believe in more than survival—when they gather around what's good, true, and lasting—they stop being a crowd and start becoming a people.

D-Faith doesn't replace the shared life of faith. It protects and strengthens it—helping preserve the witness and memory that sustain Christianity across generations.▯

So the next time someone asks what it means to live well, we don't just point to a slogan.▯

We point to a life remembered—and a community still becoming.

Chapter 25

Truth Without Ownership

Open-Source Revelation and the Future of Sacred Commons

Core Problem or Tension: For most of religious history, truth has been treated as property. Revelation has often been mediated through hierarchy. That structure helped preserve coherence—but it also created bottlenecks of control, where deviation became heresy and access came with conditions. In a decentralised age, we must ask: Can truth still be sacred if no one owns it?

What This Chapter Offers: This chapter reimagines theology as an open-source ecosystem. It proposes that sacred insight can be stewarded collaboratively—not diluted, but enriched through transparency, traceability, and ethical participation. Drawing parallels with open-source code, and examples from real-world religious projects, it suggests that the deepest truths flourish not when locked down, but when shared.

Why It Matters Now: In an era shaped by collaborative platforms and decentralised systems, a new model of faith transmission is emerging—one rooted in contribution, review, and moral coherence.

"Given enough eyeballs, all bugs are shallow."

— Eric S. Raymond

The powerful have long tried to own truth—not because it belonged to them, but because they knew it shaped the world. They sought to safeguard it through doctrine, councils, and creeds—efforts that often preserved coherence and unity, but at times also restricted access. Over the centuries, this safeguarding sometimes took the unintended shape of treating truth as property, even when the goal was to protect it. Access required a license. The result was not just control, but dependence: people could not act on what they saw without approval from those above them.

But what if truth doesn't wither when it's shared, but begins to breathe? Like open-source code, theology grows stronger when tested, reviewed, and refined. Scientists have known this for centuries—the scientific method itself relies on structured peer review. The point is not innovation for its own sake, but resilience: ideas survive precisely because they can be examined and improved.

For much of history, revelation travelled through narrow, controlled channels. A prophet spoke, priests defined and councils set boundaries. The original burst of vision and energy became formal rules and committees — which kept order but sometimes made dissent costly. In those moments, the pursuit of stability risked overshadowing the vitality that first gave the movement life.

Open revelation changes that system. Sacred knowledge, like open-source software, can be inspected, debated, and even forked without severing its roots. Peer-reviewed faith. Version control with reverence. When disagreements are logged openly, future generations inherit not only the texts but the reasoning that shaped them.

Truth without ownership does not mean theology will dissolve into chaos. Consensus can emerge when interpretations are logged, reviewed, and tested over time. The payoff is coherence: a faith resilient enough to hold many voices without silencing any of them. Disagreement, recorded faithfully, becomes a gift—giving later generations the dignity of choice and the map of how others wrestled before them.

In D-Faith, revelation lives as a shared library—open to seekers, enriched by contributors, and strengthened across time. It is tended like a commons, where wisdom grows through return and re-examination. Prophets are remembered not only because they safeguarded the story in their time, but because their words still speak—fitting patterns of goodness that continue to orient us. Reverence deepens, not when insight is locked away, but when it is carried forward collectively.

Tradition matters, too. While it anchors us it must also be given room to breathe. Sefaria's digital library places Jewish texts alongside centuries of commentary, allowing new generations to enter the conversation. Qur'an Gateway invites rigorous historical engagement with Islam's sacred text. Creative Commons liturgies circulate in Christianity, created and shared by communities themselves. These are glimpses of open theology already at work.

A wisdom commons is not immune to sabotage, yet decentralisation can resist without disorder. Steward-nodes—trusted contributors reviewing for coherence and ethical alignment—can provide stability. Alongside the safeguards long provided by faithful leadership and tradition, transparency, attribution, and auditability can now serve as complementary protections in a digital age

In such a system, a prayer, commentary, or question becomes part of a living archive, where others can learn, respond, and add their voice. The record itself becomes the theology: layered, accountable, and alive. Shared revelation trusts that God still speaks through many voices in harmony with the truth He has already entrusted to His people—and that our understanding of that truth deepens when tested.

As Eric Raymond quipped about open code, even the most complex problems become clear given enough eyes. Faith is no different. Let the truth be free—and watch it grow.

Postscript: The Pool Shark Problem

Trust is slow. It is earned in increments, through presence and patience. Bisq[1] knows this: a new buyer is capped at small trades until time proves them reliable. D-Faith knows it too: new voices are heard, but influence only deepens through continuity. The rhythm protects against the fast-talking stranger who demands trust at once.

But slowness itself can be gamed. The pool shark knows how to lose small and often, to build confidence in their weakness. Then, when the stakes rise, they strike. In networks of trust, the same temptation appears: take the small losses, play the long game, and betray when the pot is full.

This is the paradox of time-based trust: it both protects and exposes. What guards against the hasty fraud also invites the patient one. Which means a system built on continuity must add a further safeguard: **memory that is distributed**. Not one person's recollection, but a record that no one can quietly edit. If betrayal comes, it cannot be hidden. If trust is gamed, the fork remains open—continuity is preserved even if one branch proves false.

Time still builds trust. But in decentralised faith, memory makes it harder to hustle.

---

1. Bisq is a peer-to-peer, decentralised exchange where people trade Bitcoin directly with one another, without banks, intermediaries, or ID checks.

Q: *What kind of information could D-Faith actually hold on the blockchain? Could it store thoughts or prayers—or just transactions? And how would someone leave a message on it?*

A: At first glance, a blockchain seems like an unlikely place for something sacred. But look a little closer, and it reveals itself not just as a ledger of numbers—but a keeper of memory.

D-Faith wouldn't only record movement or exchange. It could preserve a whisper of a prayer, a commitment made in community, or a teaching shared across time. The technology doesn't store the prayer itself—but it can remember that it was offered, when, and by whom (if they choose). It doesn't hold heavy files or endless texts—but it can hold the proof that something was said, signed, or shared. A spiritual fingerprint, you might say. Something that says: *This happened. It's remembered.*

And yes—someone could leave a message. A single line, a reflection, or a private vow. It could be public, encrypted, or visible only to a trusted circle—depending on how the system is designed. It could live directly on the chain, or rest off-chain with only its signature embedded in the record. This means the chain stores a proof of the message—not the message itself—so sacred memory is verifiable yet private, complementing existing practices of prayer, confession, and pastoral care.

This opens a new kind of territory. A public wall that no one owns, a prayer log that can't be erased and testimony that doesn't require institutional hosting to be remembered—while remaining open to pastoral guidance and community discernment.

In D-Faith, we don't *also* need a vaulted cathedral roof to echo our beliefs—the digital layer can carry the echo alongside cathedrals and house-churches alike. The structure itself can hold those echoes. And if it's built well, it will remember—not just what we said, but that we

showed up—so faith practiced in homes, parishes, and small groups leaves a durable trace.

For a deeper exploration, read "What the Blockchain Can Store" in the Bonus Materials.

Q: *HOW DO YOU ACCOUNT FOR THOSE WHO EXPRESS FALSE VIRTUE—LEAVING MESSAGES, DEMONSTRATING PRESENCE, BUT LIVING CONTRARY TO THE IDEALS THEY LOG?*

A: There's no perfect safeguard against it. People have always found ways to display virtue without living it. Long before digital ledgers, there were public prayers offered for applause and confessions shaped for effect. The desire to be seen as good can easily outpace the desire to become good. A decentralised protocol doesn't eliminate that temptation—but it does remove the curated stage.

In D-Faith, presence alone is not a verdict; integrity is discerned in community over time. A message like *"I forgave someone today"* doesn't come with applause or accusation. It isn't a badge. It's a mark. A timestamp. A signal that something—perhaps sincere, perhaps not—was offered at a moment in time.

And yet, something else begins to emerge—not from any single act, but from the pattern of a life. The one who shows up privately, repeatedly, without feedback, begins to draw a different kind of line through the ledger—not more praised, but steadier. Over time, that pattern begins to carry its own quiet credibility.

Of course, the system itself can't know the human heart. It wasn't built to judge that—and perhaps that's part of its integrity. It doesn't pretend to read motives. It simply remembers actions. It offers a place where someone can bring their better intentions—however clumsily—without needing approval. Where another can mark their struggle without fear it will be mistaken for failure.

A false message may endure on the ledger, but it often fades within the person who wrote it. It doesn't become true just because it was recorded. But the inverse is also true: a modest, sincere message—left without fanfare, perhaps even in grief—can become a source of strength, long after the moment has passed.

In that way, D-Faith offers something subtle but significant. It is not surveillance, nor a performance arena—just the chance to witness. A way to say: *I was here. I tried. I meant this.*

And for some, that small act of permanence may be more powerful than anyone else will ever know.

Q: *Isn't The Reputation Graph Just a Social Credit Score?*

A: It's a fair concern. At a glance, the Reputation Graph might resemble a system for tracking behavior, but its nature is very different. Unlike credit systems, which are imposed, invisible, and built for control, the Reputation Graph begins with consent. Nothing is automatic. Every record emerges from voluntary connection.

What's remembered isn't a score. It's a moment—a kept promise, a repaired wrong, an act of generosity—not abstract metrics, but living memory that serves Christian formation

When someone falls short, growth is part of the record. The ledger includes the turning back, not just the falling away.

There's no reward structure, ranking, or market for appearances. We compile these records to remember—to honour the patterns of trust, repair, and integrity that shape who we become.

That difference is not just technical. It's moral—because it doesn't reward appearance, it remembers integrity, shaping how people show up, forgive, and begin again.

For a deeper exploration, read "Not a Social Credit Score" in the Bonus Materials.

Chapter 26

Permissionless Faith

The Inversion of Freedom and Risk

> "It is not the chains of others that keep us from being free. It is the chains we place upon ourselves and our refusal to walk beyond them."
>
> — Kahlil Gibran

Freedom has long been romanticised—as if liberty itself were the destination. In modern life, it's often reduced to autonomy or endless choice. But the real question is not how to become free, but how to stay free.

In D-Faith, there is no centralised priestly office or governing council within the system itself. Freedom is the default and designed to work in harmony with the teaching, pastoral care, and sacramental life of the Church where believers are already rooted. Each person is both seeker and steward: Your node is your personal place of testimony, with your discernment forming part of your daily liturgy—complementing the worship, sacraments, and discipleship offered in Christian community. Such trust is radical and heavy. Kierkegaard saw it clearly: freedom provokes dread, not because it is bad, but because it is real.

Freedom Without Formation

Freedom without formation drifts. In the modern West, *negative liberty* has dominated—the freedom from shame, tradition, or duty. But Isaiah Berlin reminded us that *positive liberty*—the freedom to become—requires scaffolding, rhythm, and companionship. It is not simply the

absence of constraint; it is the presence of conditions that help us grow into what we were meant to be. Without these, freedom can turn to aimlessness or isolation. With them, it becomes the soil in which courage, generosity, and wisdom take root. True liberty is not only the power to choose, but the power to choose well, shaped by practices, mentors, and communities that make the good both visible and possible.

Conscience does not grow in isolation; it deepens through memory, repetition, and the presence of others who walk with us. If D-Faith is to offer lasting freedom, it must also cultivate formation: voluntary rites of passage, shared rhythms, and spaces of accountability. Freedom becomes meaningful only when there is something worth becoming.

The Sacred Is Not Safe

In *The Lion, the Witch and the Wardrobe*, when Lucy asks if Aslan is safe, Mr. Beaver laughs: "*Safe? Who said anything about safe? 'Course he isn't safe. But he's good. He's the King, I tell you.*"

Lewis was naming something ancient—that what is truly good often unsettles before it comforts. The sacred doesn't promise to leave our lives neatly arranged; it upends them. It binds us to people we might not choose, asks questions we'd rather avoid, and exposes loyalties we didn't know we had.

In Scripture and history alike, encounters with the sacred rarely ended in comfort—they ended in new paths, new risks, and sometimes new enemies. Moses came down the mountain with law and a fractured people. Mary said yes to God and was whispered about for the rest of her life.

D-Faith inherits this pattern. It's not designed to wrap faith in bubble-wrap, but to make space where conviction can be lived out in full view. That visibility will test us: it can bring support, but it can also provoke resistance. The sacred will not guarantee safety—but it will offer something far better: the chance to be transformed in ways comfort never could.

Why Many Will Refuse

D-Faith will not suit everyone. Genuine freedom is a heavy burden to bear—it asks for both belief and the willingness to live with its consequences. Some will continue to look for pastoral leaders to follow and rituals to lean on—often within their local church—and that may be their entry point into D-Faith's shared record. Others may find the burden too much and return to older forms. Yet many will discover, over time, that they can carry more than they imagined—not because they already have the answers, but because they are learning to shoulder the questions themselves.

Conclusion

We like to imagine our chains were placed there by others. It's harder to admit how many we've chosen for ourselves.

Spiritual freedom has never depended on permission. It begins with resolve—the courage to hold fast to our convictions, taking personal responsibility for living them out, while staying connected to the wider Body of Christ. It is the choice to follow conscience over the ease of avoiding conflict—the relief of not having to face anxiety, risk, or consequence.

Some will choose safety. Others will wait for clearer voices or stronger leaders before stepping forward. But the remnant will not wait. Something within them refuses to be still—they must begin to build.

Gibran's reminder holds: the deepest chains are often the ones we fasten on ourselves. To walk beyond them is the first act of real faith.

Chapter 27

Love as Law

The Moral Operating System of D-Faith

Core Problem or Tension: Most systems—religious, legal, or social—rely on authority to keep people in line. In a decentralised faith, there's no hierarchy to enforce compliance. So what holds it together? What anchors it when no one's in charge?

What This Chapter Offers: This chapter explores a law central to Christianity—one rooted in love. Not love as sentiment, but as a deliberate, voluntary alignment with what is good. It proposes that love, rightly understood, can act as the moral protocol of a decentralised spiritual system. Drawing from scripture, moral philosophy, blockchain consensus, and restorative practices, it outlines how D-Faith can remain ethically coherent without institutional enforcement.

Why It Matters Now: In a polarized world, love—as a freely chosen, clearly lived principle—may be the only force powerful enough to unite without dominating. This chapter offers a path forward: a logic that inspires trust, belonging, and moral clarity.

> *"Power without love is reckless and abusive, and love without power is sentimental and anemic."*
>
> — Martin Luther King Jr.

The Limits of Command

Throughout history, God has given moral direction both directly—through the Law, the Prophets, and Christ Himself—and through the structures of His people, including councils, pastors, and courts. These have preserved order and often transformed lives. Yet at times, when the focus shifted toward rule-keeping without conversion of the heart, the call to love God and neighbour could be obscured. D-Faith seeks to serve as one more means of rekindling that love in the Church and beyond. As Alasdair MacIntyre observed, our moral language has drifted into abstraction—"duty," "rights," "justice"—words unmoored from shared purpose. We behave, but we don't believe. We conform, but we don't belong.

Love as the Deep Protocol

When asked the greatest commandment, Jesus didn't give a rule—He pointed to a relationship: *"Love the Lord your God with all your heart... and love your neighbour as yourself"* (Matthew 22:37–40). In that moment, the logic of morality shifted. Law was no longer external decree but an orientation of the heart.

Rightly understood, love is not sentiment but alignment. It binds like gravity—subtle, constant, and inescapable. In decentralised terms, the protocol is the architecture that holds everything together without hierarchy or fear. Love doesn't need to be enforced; because it draws us, builds trust, and sustains coherence.

D-Faith must inherit this: a moral architecture rooted in love—binding enough to hold, free enough to inspire.

Consensus Without Coercion

Blockchains verify truth through consensus. Each node participates, each voice matters, and integrity grows through shared responsibility.

The same pattern holds for moral life: meaning emerges when commitments are chosen and sustained. In early Christianity, love was the proof of faith; Paul insisted that even prophecy and sacrifice were hollow without it (1 Corinthians 13).

Accountability Through Belonging

Within D-Faith's decentralised design, there is no central priestly office or governing council to enforce discipline. This does not replace the role of pastoral leadership or Church discipline where believers are rooted in a local fellowship. Instead, it offers an additional framework for addressing harm through restorative means—particularly for those on the margins or outside traditional structures—while remaining open to partnership with the wider Body of Christ. Communities already offer models. Quakers use clearness committees for discernment. Recovery groups assign sponsors to guide moral repair. These practices show that accountability can be restorative: not punishment from above, but correction through care. In D-Faith, harming another damages the network of trust. Restoration is a call back to belonging, not a sentence of exclusion.

A Moral Operating System

For love to function as law, it must be structured:

— **Voluntary Alignment**: Love coerced isn't love.

— **Transparent Action**: Integrity is visible, not performative.

— **Witnessed Integrity**: Moral acts gain strength when seen and remembered.

— **Immutable Trace**: Lives shaped by love leave records of faithfulness.

— **Forks with Grace**: Even divergence must honour the bond of love.

From Rights to Responsibilities

Modern culture exalts rights but forgets obligations. Viktor Frankl warned that freedom without responsibility is arbitrariness. In D-Faith, freedom is sacred not because it permits anything, but because it directs us toward the good. To love freely is to bind oneself to what is sacred—and to act accordingly.

Law as love: This is the inheritance D-Faith seeks to help carry forward, alongside the historic witness of the Church. Not replacing godly leadership or fellowship, but complementing them with tools that make love visible, remembered, and lived. The goal is not to abolish hierarchy where it serves faithfully, but to ensure that love remains the deepest protocol guiding both Church and decentralised life.

King's words return as a reminder: power needs love, and love needs power.

Chapter 28

The Genesis Document

Core Problem or Tension: Movements without origin drift. Origins without integrity corrode. Every faith needs a beginning—but in the decentralised age, how do you establish one without hierarchy, gatekeeping, or revisionist history? How do you create a sacred starting point that welcomes contribution, resists corruption, and retains coherence across divergence?

What This Chapter Offers: An exploration of the Genesis Document: a public, inspectable, forkable foundation for D-Faith. It outlines its structure, spiritual rationale, technological underpinnings, and how it may be distributed, adopted, and evolve. Drawing from scripture, open-source culture, and covenantal traditions; a way to begin—transparent and transcendent.

Why It Matters Now: Movements that cannot name their origin are vulnerable to manipulation. Those that cannot evolve are brittle. The Genesis Document offers both integrity and flexibility—embedding first principles without pretending to be final truth. It gives early communities something to orient by, build from, and return to—as a true and steady compass.

"In the beginning was the Word."

—John 1:1

> *"We the People of the United States, in Order to form a more perfect Union, establish Justice, insure domestic Tranquility, provide for the common defence, promote the general Welfare, and secure the Blessings of Liberty to ourselves and our Posterity, do ordain and establish this Constitution for the United States of America."*
>
> Preamble to The U.S. Constitution

That preamble wasn't only a political statement; it was a protocol. It declared what mattered, who mattered, and how decisions would be carried forward. If every principle of D-Faith began from such a foundation, it might not yield perfection, but it would lean toward justice, mercy, and truth that no one could lock away.

Every spiritual movement has a moment of origin—Moses on Sinai, Muhammad in the cave, Siddhartha beneath the tree. These remain sacred to billions, and for good reason—they anchor communities of faith. Yet historically, they were mediated through trusted authority and preserved by hierarchical stewardship, which in some cases also limited direct access for the wider community.

> *We, the contributors to this Genesis Document, this shared chain of meaning, establish a forkable, inspectable foundation for the recording of sacred insight, to preserve traceable lineage, enable transparent accountable participation, support interpretive continuity, and sustain a living incorruptible record of faith, offered in trust for those who seek, contribute, and remember, for all generations to come.*
>
> — Preamble to the Genesis Document

D-Faith begins differently, not as a new revelation replacing what came before, but as a public, inspectable, traceable covenant designed

to complement the witness of the Church—born in openness so that faith can be strengthened and remembered in our own time. Let us call it the *Genesis Document.* A spiritual code: part declaration, part covenant, part design. Holy because it tells the truth about itself—its origins, limits, and invitation.

The question is not simply "*what will this document say?*" but "*why will it matter?* " Because the opening layer of any system reveals its heart. Constitutions, creeds, and even software all betray what their builders valued most. If the foundation of D-Faith is to hold, it must be more than functional. It must be faithful—to something enduring and incorruptible.

Precedents and InspirationsWhat

The Genesis Document has ancestors worth remembering:

— The **U.S. Constitution (1787)**: concise, intent-driven, amendable.

— The **Tao Te Ching (c. 400 BC)**: elegant, cryptic, endlessly generative.

— **Luther's 95 Theses (1517)**: disruptive, morally urgent, catalytic.

— The **Bitcoin Whitepaper (2008)**: transparent, distributed, trustless by design.

D-Faith would learn from Satoshi: anonymity over celebrity, refusal to profit, transparency as integrity. It would echo covenantal theology: mutual responsibility, voluntary alignment. And it would resist what Shoshana Zuboff calls *surveillance capitalism*—transparent but never extractive.

Functions of the Genesis Document

At its heart, the document serves five functions:

1. **Declare First Principles** — truth, compassion, covenant, mutual dignity.

2. **Outline Structural Commitments** — how consensus is achieved, how memory is kept.

3. **Define Its Limitations** — this is Version 1.0, open to revision in light, never in secret.

4. **Invite Participation** — every reader is a potential node, contributor, or steward.

5. **Commit to Incorruptibility** — time-stamped, hashed, forkable; it cannot be secretly erased.

It is not a creed, or a sales pitch. It is a covenant of trust.

The Root Layer: Who Is God?

If the Genesis Document matters at all, it must anchor itself in what is least debatable. Across centuries of theology, disagreement abounds—but some declarations endure:

— *God is One.* "Hear, O Israel: the Lord our God, the Lord is one" (Deut. 6:4). One source, no rival claimants.

— *God is Just.* "The Lord is a God of justice" (Isa. 30:18). Not arbitrary, not partial. Justice as nature, not mood.

— *God is Compassionate and Faithful.* "Slow to anger, abounding in love" (Ex. 34:6). God doesn't just demand faith—He embodies it.

— *God is Love.* "Whoever does not love does not know God" (1 John 4:8). Not "has" love. *Is* love.

— *God is Spirit.* "God is spirit, and his worshipers must worship in spirit and truth" (John 4:24). No walls, robes, or licenses can contain Him.

— *God shows no partiality.* (Acts 10:34). No VIP tier. No elite elect.

This is not lowest-common-denominator theology. It is a floor—an irreducible consensus that — God is unified, just, loving, and non-coercive.

Ethical Safeguards: Integrity as Code

Every system needs red lines. Law has constitutions, blockchain has hashes, and faith has conscience. If D-Faith has none, it becomes another ideology for hire.

It is unlikely that the Genesis Document will begin from first principles. To discard the wisdom of the past would be an act of hubris—an arrogance blind to the tests of time. It will draw from scriptures and moral traditions that have endured millennia, precisely because their survival is itself a witness. They carry the refinements of struggle and testing, and remind us that we cannot shortcut what only generations can prove trustworthy.

— **No manipulation in God's name.** "You shall not misuse the name of the Lord your God" (Ex. 20:7).

— **Love as the final test.** "The entire law is fulfilled in keeping this one command: 'Love your neighbor as yourself'" (Gal. 5:14).

— **Openness without relativism.** "Test everything. Hold fast to what is good" (1 Thess. 5:21).

— **No monetisation of grace.** Jesus overturning the money changers (Matt. 21:12).

— **Humility before mystery.** "Now we see through a glass, darkly" (1 Cor. 13:12).

These are not aspirations. They are consensus signals. Without them, the system corrupts.

The "Do Not Touch" List

Some lines must be unalterable:

— Do not shame or exclude in the name of truth.

— Do not hard-code doctrines that love and humility cannot verify.

— Do not restrict salvation or belonging.

— Do not license access to God.

— Do not claim to speak *for* God, only *with* God.

Immutable does not mean inflexible. Forking is possible, but these anchors remain.

Universal Anchors Across Traditions

Sacred texts across civilizations echo the same moral DNA:

— *Do not kill. Do not steal. Do not bear false witness* (Exod. 20).

— *So God created mankind in his image* (Gen. 1:27).

— *Do unto others as you would have them do unto you* (Matt. 7:12, also Confucius, Buddhism, Islam).

— *Act justly, love mercy, walk humbly* (Mic. 6:8).

— *Blessed are the peacemakers* (Matt. 5:9).

— *No compulsion in religion* (Qur'an 2:256).

— The *Noble Eightfold Path* (Buddhism).

Not all will agree on every phrase, but together they show the bedrock of conscience that survives culture, empire, and reform.

Structure: Three Parts, One Posture

1. **Statement of Meaning** — why it exists, what it honors, and refuses to be.
    - Truth is not owned, only witnessed.
    - Mystery is boundary, not weakness.
    - No one is too small to participate, and no authority is too great to escape scrutiny.
2. **Covenant of Participation** — mechanics of belonging: roles of witness, interpreter, contributor; consensus through logged participation; transparent amendment.
3. **Declaration of Intent** — this is Version 1.0. Imperfect, but incorruptible. Never changed silently or alone.

The form mirrors open-source systems, yet its spirit is bound by shared promise rather than profit.

Anchored but Alive

The Ten Commandments are not merely ancient laws but civilizational axioms: Don't murder, don't steal, don't lie. Their relevance is not rigidity but resonance with human trust. The Genesis Document must function the same way—open to commentary and iteration, yet unshakable at its moral core.

John's gospel might have opened with its own preamble: *"In the beginning was the Word, and to the Word we now bear witness. What we have known in love, we preserve... that the life made known to us may not pass away, but live on in those who seek and those yet to be born."*

That is the tone: humble yet clear, grounded in conviction.

Technological Properties

To matter, the Genesis Document must carry technological and theological integrity.

— **Immutable:** no silent edits. Every version visible.

— **Provenant:** clear lineage from the original hash.

— **Decentralised:** no single host. Stored across nodes.

— **Participatory:** anyone can mirror, propose, or annotate.

It may live on IPFS, Git, or other distributed systems. It can be printed, sung, embedded in metadata, or read aloud in rituals. The form may vary, but the integrity cannot.

Forking With Fidelity

Forking in D-Faith is moral iteration, not convenience. When conscience demands divergence, a fork must:

— Reference the parent document.

— Record its hash.

—Justify the change.

The Torah was not customisable, the Beatitudes were not a buffet, and the Buddha's path was not optional. Traditions endure not because they please but because they bind.

In Summary

John begins his Gospel with words that echo like a genesis of their own: *"In the beginning was the Word, and the Word was with God, and the Word was God"* (John 1:1). That opening was not only theology—it was testimony. The Word was not locked away in a temple or scroll; it was spoken into time, remembered by witnesses, carried by the community, and made flesh among us.

In the same spirit, the Genesis Document is intended to be witnessed. It is meant to live among those who will read it, fork it, test it, and pass it on. Its power lies in its faithfulness—an incorruptible record that says: this is where we began, what we carried, and what we refused to let be lost. If the Gospel of John tells us that the Word was the light that darkness could not overcome, then the Genesis Document is one small attempt to mirror that claim in our own age: a light no council can extinguish, no hierarchy can misuse, and no generation can erase—ensuring the wisdom entrusted to God's people can be preserved alongside the living witness of the Church. This record will insist that memory is sacred, and that truth, when shared, grows stronger.

Yet its strength lies not only in its stories, but in its purpose. The Genesis Document is a root layer—a covenantal ledger of first principles. It encodes ethical anchors: life is sacred, love is the test, and truth must remain transparent. It names foundational axioms: Faith must allow faithful re-examination, no authority is beyond humble accountability, and mystery itself remains essential. It also binds core commitments: consensus with integrity, participation without gatekeeping, and stewardship not ownership.

This is robust scaffolding built from wisdom that has endured millennia, tested by time in ways no single generation could reproduce. To

inscribe them now is to admit that conscience, like code, needs a reference layer—a point all can return to when disputes arise or memory begins to fade.

The Genesis Document is not the Word made flesh, but it can aspire to mirror the same role: a beginning that orients, a foundation that holds, a light by which those who walk may see more clearly.

***Q:** How would I actually leave a message in D-Faith? If I wanted to record something permanent—what would that process look like?*

A: It begins with a decision: what are you trying to preserve?

A simple line—like "I forgave her today"—can be written directly into the blockchain, provided it's short enough. That message, once committed, is distributed across the network, time-stamped, and tamper-evident. It's not hosted by a company or stored in a personal journal—it becomes part of the shared record. Not to be evaluated or ranked, but to exist. To persist.

If your message is longer or something you'd prefer to keep private, it can be stored off-chain in a decentralised file system. The blockchain itself will hold only a fingerprint—a cryptographic hash that proves the message existed, intact, at a particular moment in time. You can choose to share the content or not. The proof remains either way.

There's no login. No moderator. You sign the message with a private key—your proof of authorship. That's it. You don't need permission to write. The act of writing *is* the signal.

The system maintains order—limiting message size, validating signatures, resisting spam—but stays open-ended. You could write once, or return over the years. Each trace builds upon the last.

What you leave behind won't get lost in a feed. It won't be deleted when the terms change. It won't be monetized. It will remain there, anchored and immutable, because you chose to mark it.

That's how D-Faith operates—by encoding memory in infrastructure, and removing barriers to participation—so that believers and seekers alike can record and preserve acts of faith alongside the witness already carried by the Church.

For a deeper exploration, read "Leaving a Trace: How to Store a Message" in the Bonus Materials.

Chapter 29

First Contact

— How D-Faith Begins in a Single Life

Core Problem or Tension: Faith often begins with a feeling—subtle, nameless. Yet most systems speak to the already convinced. They expect fluency, commitment, alignment. But many today carry a hunger they've lost the vocabulary to describe, unsure how to begin.

What This Chapter Offers: Tracing a first encounter with D-Faith through Mateo, an ordinary man, we glimpse how sacred rhythm might reach someone in practice, without requiring immediate belief—just their presence, repeated action, and place to begin.

Why It Matters Now: Spiritual longing may be less often articulated nowadays, maybe harder to name. In a world of noise, people want something that feels real, that connects with them at a deep emotional level. D-Faith can meet them there, not with all the answers, but with rhythm. This is how it might begin.

"Go sit in your cell, and your cell will teach you everything"[1]

— Desert Fathers

---

1. Early Christian monks who withdrew into the Egyptian desert during the 3rd–5th centuries. Linked to *Abba Moses* or *Abba Arsenius.*

Before there is code, covenant, or creed, there is someone waking up to an ordinary day—aware that something vital has gone missing, but unable to articulate it. No lightning bolt, or conversion moment. Just the uneasy sense that life has become thinner, and that meaning—if it still exists—has drifted out of reach.

If D-Faith matters, it must start here, with a single human life and the smallest possible step toward living differently.

An Invitation Without Strings

Mateo, a bus driver in his forties, finds a plain white card at his local café:

"You are not alone. There is a way to live that is sacred, decentralised, and real. Ask me about D-Faith."

That night, the QR code leads to a page with no login, no catch—just:

"Act with integrity, even when unseen.

Honour what transcends you.

Repair what you break."

Daily prompts ask: "*Who will you treat with patience today?*" And, at day's end, "*Where did you fall short?*"

In a culture drowning in noise and constant demands for attention, a clean, anonymous starting point is rare. By offering no accounts, tracking, or demands, the first encounter with D-Faith earns trust before it asks for commitment.

A Personal Anchor

If the practice takes root, a user can generate a private key—a cryptographic signature that remembers them without identifying them.

Spiritual growth often falters when there is nothing to hold it in place. This key provides an immutable personal record—kept locally and shared only with consent—so that each person carries a living moral trail that belongs entirely to them, not an institution.

Technology in the Background

Under the surface, blockchain ensures incorruptibility, but the experience feels like a private journal with optional public witness.

Faith systems that rely solely on fragile institutions or central servers can disappear overnight. D-Faith is designed to survive without them—able to function offline, backed up on paper, and adaptable in the face of censorship—so the practice can continue even in disruption.

The First Week

Users try three commitments, log reflections, and exchange brief signals with a small, anonymous circle:

"I forgave someone today."

"I stayed silent when I should have spoken."

At week's end, they're simply asked: "*Do you want to keep going?*"

Because there is no threat, no guilt, and no cost to stepping away, participation is sustained by genuine desire rather than pressure—and that makes staying more meaningful.

Practice at its Core

Over time, rituals may emerge—candles before reflection, annotating sacred texts privately, contributing to prayer chains. Every seven days, a deeper question arrives:

"Where were you tempted to take the easy way out?"

Good intentions fade without regular renewal. These small, repeated prompts keep the work alive, strengthening the moral muscle a little at a time.

It's for Them

One day, they catch themselves pausing before speaking sharply, listening more than talking. Small changes begin to feel natural rather than forced.

That's when they know it's for them—not because they have artificially cloaked themselves in a new identity, but because they have become noticeably more patient, grounded, and intentional.

D-Faith does not replace belief—or the witness and life of the Church—it supports them, offering scaffolding where tradition cannot presently reach or where it welcomes renewal. The beginning is simple: intention, curiosity, and the hope that something sacred still wants to be found.

The Desert Fathers knew that a cell was never just four walls. It was the place where you confronted yourself—where silence became a teacher and stillness stripped away pretense. In the same way, D-Faith begins in the smallest of cells: a moment of private intention, an unseen act of repair, a line you write primarily for yourself.

If it teaches you anything, it's that sacred change doesn't wait for perfect conditions. It begins in the life you already have and asks only that you remain long enough for those ageless forces to work on you—just as they shaped your ancestors, and as they will shape those yet to come.

Chapter 30

Beyond Evangelism —

The Architecture of Invitation

Core Problem or Tension: Evangelism, as traditionally practiced, often presumes superiority. It implies a separation: the enlightened versus the ignorant. But in a decentralised spiritual age, this model alienates. How do we invite others in without reverting to coercion, manipulation, or noise?

What This Chapter Offers: A reframing of spiritual outreach as an architecture of invitation rooted in visibility, openness, and consent. How witness, ritual, and covenant can be encoded into the very structure of D-Faith, making faith discoverable without relying on persuasion. It introduces the *Reputation Graph* and, at its heart, the *Soulful Pseudonym*.

Why It Matters Now: Today everyone is selling something—often themselves. Institutions sell belief, influencers sell authenticity. In this climate, trust must be earned. Lives of quiet integrity can shift the world without ever raising a voice—and invites us to think more like hosts than preachers.

"It is no use walking anywhere to preach unless our walking is our preaching."
— Attributed in "Little Flowers of St. Francis" (Fioretti), 14th century

There was a time when monasteries sheltered the weary before they questioned their beliefs. Bread, warmth, and silence came before doctrine. D-Faith, though digital and dispersed, must carry that same DNA.

A monastery's walls once spoke reverence; now, an app can do the same. Digital spaces can be open porches—low-barrier, serene, generous in tone. No pop-ups. No pressure. Interfaces should reflect grace, not commerce. The design, cadence, and rituals must be beautiful enough to linger in memory. That beauty is part of the welcome—what is worth remembering is worth returning to.

From Conversion to Co-Creation

Traditional religion often asks for belief before belonging. D-Faith complements the historic witness of the Church by offering a path where people can belong before they fully believe. Contribute first, conviction follows—so that what begins here can, in time, strengthen their life of faith within the wider Body of Christ. Like blockchain's peer nodes, participation shapes the system itself. A reflection, a shared struggle, an improvement to the protocol—these acts don't happen on the threshold; they *are* the threshold.

In the digital wilderness, noise doesn't persuade—coherence does. D-Faith grows through the steady presence of people whose lives radiate kindness, responsibility, and reverence. Like the early Christians described as "a peculiar people," they draw others not by argument, but by example.

Liturgies Without Walls

Every faith has rhythms—Sabbaths, fasts, prayers. In D-Faith, liturgy is open-source ritual: daily check-ins with conscience, public commitments to others, humility built into feedback loops. Interfaces make virtue visible, like blockchain's traceable actions.

A DAO might open with collective silence. A node might track acts of generosity—not to build ego, but to encourage habits that reshape the giver. These rhythms spread because they are beautiful *and* transformative.

In D-Faith, entry begins with consent—fully informed, freely given, publicly logged. The covenant is explicit, like a smart contract for the soul:

— Commit to truthfulness, even when costly.

— Uphold dignity in speech and silence.

— Seek reconciliation before retribution.

— Accept correction and correct with care.

No hidden clauses. You see it before you sign. You bind yourself with your name—literal or pseudonymous—and that act becomes the bond.

When Failure Invites Repair

Shame isolates, but compassionate accountability restores. In D-Faith, falling short results in a call to repair: mediated reflection, recommitment, and community support. Its architecture makes this possible—logs that remember not just what broke but what healed. The call to live by that standard still remains, except now, there's a way home.

The Reputation Graph: Sacred Memory at Scale[1]

In the surveillance age, reputation is often reduced to a fragile performance. D-Faith envisions something better—a *ledger of unseen acts*, preserved through earned trust in a decentralised web. At its heart is

1. Functioning across a large network, or ecosystem.

the soulful pseudonym: an identity that hides the face but reveals the character.

Attestations might read:

— "She kept her promise."

— "He returned to reconcile."

— "They stood by the vulnerable."

Over time, these small recognitions form a trust-fingerprint—not for ranking, but for remembrance.

The Soulful Pseudonym

Privacy remains intact. History accrues. A soulful pseudonym says: *Judge me not by my appearance, but by my actions.* Trust grows through patterns of integrity: a decade of reconciliations, contributions, and care is almost impossible to fake.

Proof Without Surveillance

Identity is verified through a cryptographic keypair—your "soulprint." Every act you sign confirms continuity without revealing your name. Multi-identity abuse is discouraged not through policing, but because memory accrues slowly, cannot be bought, and is bound to moral commitments in the Genesis Document.

Guardrails Against Manipulation

To keep trust from becoming vanity:

— Reputation grows or fades with time.

— Diverse relationships count more than insular ones.

— Growth after failure is weighted higher than a perfect mask.

Curated Transparency

Not every act needs to be public. The system surfaces signals, not noise:

— Acts of reconciliation
— Votes grounded in love
— Patterns of long-term care

Each is verifiable, but no one must scroll endlessly to feel the texture of a person's or community's witness.

Pilgrim Stone

Consider Pilgrim Stone. No one knows her real name. But her record holds endorsements from across the world: "She listened when no one else would." "She stayed in the hard moments." She's never spoken on a stage, but her witness is known.

Meeting her, you don't see cold, objective metrics. You see:

"*Endorsed by 12 long-term nodes for humility in conflict and generosity under pressure.*"

You can read the witness logs if you want. But you already know enough: this is someone whose walk is their preaching.

The Franciscan spirit lives on here—not in friaries or robes, but in a network of lives that preach by how they walk. The welcome is not a door you pass through once, but a pattern you return to. The architecture remembers. The people remember. And in that memory, there is still bread for the hungry, shelter for the weary, and a place where the walk *is* the witness.

Chapter 31

Why They Show Up

— Motivation Without Money

Core Problem or Tension: Without formal structures or authority, continuity can fray. The challenge is not attendance, but authentic presence—an enduring connection that forms through rhythm, memory, and meaning. Some systems thrive without rewards, rules, or recognition. People return because something essential resonates.

What This Chapter Offers: This chapter explores how participation becomes belonging through small, repeated acts. It shows how people root themselves in systems that reflect their values, hold their memories, and offer a place to be known—even anonymously.

Why It Matters Now: In a volatile world people seek anchors. When a system invites expression, holds what's offered, and allows presence to accumulate, it becomes more than a platform—it becomes a place to live a life that leaves a trace.

> *Real generosity toward the future lies in giving all to the present.*
>
> —Albert Camus, Notebooks: 1935–1951

Why People Build Without Pay

What makes people keep showing up to something they're not paid for?▯
In a decentralised spiritual system, there are no salaries, no titles to climb a ladder toward, no audience to impress. So why would anyone commit to it for years—maybe a lifetime?

Because human beings are wired for meaning.

Because permanence in what we love feels like an act of justice.

Because contributing to something bigger than ourselves transforms strangers into neighbours.

Antoine de Saint-Exupéry offered a clue: "*If you want to build a ship, don't drum up people to collect wood... teach them to long for the immensity of the sea.*" In D-Faith, the "sea" is the assurance that what matters will endure — that baptisms, vows, acts of forgiveness, prayers, and testimonies will outlast their makers.

This is why Wikipedia still grows, volunteer fire brigades stand ready and community gardens are restored in cities their caretakers don't own. They join not because someone pays them, but because the culture mirrors something inside them: a truth they want to keep alive.

In D-Faith, logging a baptism is more than storing data — it's an act of witness. Recording a vow is more than keeping minutes — it's saying *this will still be here when I'm gone.* Participation becomes identity. Identity becomes devotion.

Sometimes people participate not out of mission, but because a place feels like home. Like contributors to Wikipedia or volunteers in city gardens, they join because the culture reflects something they believe in. In D-Faith, belonging grows from shared intention, not gatekeeping. Over time, a network of spiritual neighbours forms—bounded only by the choice to keep showing up.

Permanence as Dignity

Historians know the fragility of memory. Stone tablets erode, paper burns, digital files decay. Centralised platforms make deletion easy and permanence rare. But decentralised ledgers multiply themselves across continents, building resilience into the record.

That resilience matters when memory is contested. A grandmother's conversion story, a child's first prayer, the moment someone forgave—these become part of an incorruptible archive. No council can rewrite them. No algorithm can hide them. In places where trust is thin, permanence isn't just technical—it restores a dignity the soul longs for.

Designing for Devotion

Participation rarely happens by accident. It must be woven into the design. The protocol should declare its moral anchors, offer clear and welcoming paths for contribution, and help people feel that what they offer is recognised and valued. When the architecture itself honours presence, even the smallest acts become part of something enduring.

When a system allows presence to accumulate and honours small acts as sacred, participation becomes a form of devotion. Belief becomes infrastructure. And people return because it feels more permanent than the shifting world outside.

Generosity to the Future

If Bitcoin proved money could be decentralised, D-Faith dares to ask: can the work of preserving and sharing meaning be decentralised too—in a way that strengthens and complements the mission to carry the gospel into every generation?

People won't come only because it's useful. They'll come because it holds what they love and lets them place it into the bedrock of time. In

that sense, every act of participation is already a gift to those who will come after.

In such a system, participation is not a feature. It's a calling. And those who answer it will be living what Camus meant: giving all to the present so that the future may still have something worth remembering.

Chapter 32

A Rule of Life for the Decentralised Age

Core Problem or Tension: In a world saturated with autonomy and acceleration, many feel spiritually scattered. Without shared rhythms or sacred anchors, freedom becomes disorientation. How can a decentralised spiritual movement offer coherence without coercion?

What This Chapter Offers: How a "Rule of Life" can take form in a decentralised age—not as a command, but as a collective rhythm. It examines the power of repeated practices to shape character, foster belonging, and ground belief in time.

Why It Matters Now: Belief without embodiment fades. Without shared ways of living, even the most inspired visions struggle to last. This chapter invites readers to consider rhythm as sacred infrastructure—a gentle structure for holding what matters when so much feels untethered.

> "You do not rise to the level of your goals. You fall to the level of your systems,"
>
> —James Clear, Atomic Habits

In monastic life, a "Rule of Life"[1] was not a cage but a daily rhythm. St. Benedict's rule shaped the day with prayer, work, silence, and rest. Unquestioned repetition carried the sacred into ordinary time, transforming routine into devotion.

Today, the binding power of such rules has faded, yet the longing for spiritual rhythm has not. In an age of constant choice and noise, many drift in fatigue—driven but directionless. Philosopher Byung-Chul Han calls this our "fatigue society": overstimulated, yet undernourished in meaning. Rhythm is not a luxury here—it's a lifeline.

Tech Shabbat

In D-Faith, no central authority issues a universal rule. Yet the need remains: to align our days with what we claim to believe. As the Benedictines sanctified the ordinary, decentralised communities can create their own shared rhythms—local, adaptable, and forkable.

Some already do. Journalist Tiffany Shlain's "Tech Shabbat" is a day each week without devices—what began as an experiment became sacred because it preserved what mattered. In D-Faith, one node might keep sunset reflections, another might gather for a moment of shared silence.

In the historic Church, behaviour was often shaped by the conviction that God—and the community of faith He gathers—were always present to witness our lives. In D-Faith, there is no centralised human authority watching, yet every act still leaves a trace. Contributions, such as open-source code or a Wikipedia edit history, are transparent and attributable. The permanence of the record becomes the accountability.

---

1. In monastic terms, a **Rule of Life** is a written framework that sets out how members of a religious community will live, pray, and work together in pursuit of their spiritual calling. Today, some laypeople adopt a personal or community "rule of life" as a spiritual discipline—a voluntary pattern of practices that help them live intentionally according to their faith, without necessarily being in a monastery.

This traceability isn't for punishment—it's for trust. Public vows, visible acts of service, and reconciliation logs build ethical credibility. Forkable liturgies can show who contributed, where they diverged, and why. In this way, proof-of-practice becomes not a system of control, but a mirror for reflection.

The Anchor Practice

Significant change rarely starts big. One repeated act—daily reflection, gratitude logging, a whispered commitment before sleep—can become the hinge for more profound transformation. As James Clear writes, "Every action is a vote for the type of person you wish to become."

In D-Faith, a Rule of Life is less a fixed decree and more a shared protocol—modular, evolving, responsive. Its core principles—rhythm, reverence, service, truthfulness, communal trust—remain constant, even as local variations and seasonal practices emerge.

Early monastic rules were sung, embroidered, and memorised. They endured because they were beautiful. In D-Faith, beauty might live in the interface of a shared journal, the design of a visual calendar, or the cadence of reminders that feel like invitations, not demands. Beauty sustains attention, and what is worth remembering is worth returning to.

Why It Matters

Without rhythm, decentralised communities risk drifting into the same fragmentation that unravels so much of modern life. A Rule of Life—adapted for a networked age—anchors action in shared intention. It creates patterns strong enough to carry meaning forward, even when belief wavers or leadership changes.

These patterns become the vessel that holds trust. Protocol gives them form. Together, they allow holiness to become not a distant ideal, but the atmosphere in which ordinary lives are lived.

We don't need more pressure. We need patterns strong enough to keep what matters from slipping away.

Rhythm is the vessel.

Protocol is the scaffold.

Trust is the fruit.

— *Holiness* is the atmosphere that forms when all three align.

Ultimately, we rarely rise to the height of our aspirations—we return to the shape of our daily systems. Build the right rhythm, and it will carry you further than intention alone ever could.

Chapter 33

Heirs of the Protocol:

Inheritance and Succession

Core Problem or Tension: The West severed its connection to the transcendent with surgical precision—and called it enlightenment. What good is a belief system if it dies with us and what can it achieve if it re-kindles transcendence? Can faith—dispersed, decentralised, and freely chosen—still survive the slow erosion of memory, or will it fade?

What This Chapter Offers: A reflection on how sacred responsibility moves between generations and across new participation. It considers the formative work of passing forward memory, shaping moral imagination, and preparing others to contribute with integrity to something still unfolding.

Why It Matters Now: What we build now only endures if others can step into it and carry it forward. This chapter speaks to the urgency of preparing future contributors to see themselves within the story, and to shape it through memory, love, and the kind of courage that shows itself through action. Also, the consequences of forgetting. Let us rekindle transcendence in the West.

"The past is never dead. It's not even past."

— William Faulkner

Imagine your child asking, "*What does this chain mean, and why is my name on it?*" Then watching them find your name, too. What did you add, what did you verify, and what did you stand for? Every act of inheritance is a test of faith — not only in God, but in each other. No system, however elegant, survives unless the next generation believes it's worth carrying forward.

Memory Binds

Every faith worth its name is, at heart, an act of memory. The Shema, the Lord's Prayer, and ancestral stories — all are ritualised ways of remembering who we are and what matters most. The greatest danger to any sacred system isn't heresy. It's *amnesia.*

If D-Faith is to last beyond the present moment, it must become a story that outlives its tellers — one that can be questioned, reshaped, and re-verified but never forgotten.

Decentralised ≠ Disconnected

Even without centralised oversight from bishops, councils, or headquarters, it is shared coordinates—principles, protocols, and stories—that hold people together. These anchors can stand alongside the enduring witness of the Church, offering ways for each generation to navigate by them, even when the terrain shifts.

As Lawrence Lessig wrote of "*code as law,*" architecture can shape behaviour as powerfully as written rules. So too, the architecture of D-Faith becomes a moral compass: the structure teaches as much as the story. The protocol is the scripture.

Rites of Passage in a Networked World

Every tradition has a moment when the child becomes an heir — bar mitzvah, baptism, confirmation. In D-Faith, these moments may look different. Instead of reciting creeds, a young person might contribute

to the shared chain — a truth told, a reconciliation recorded, an act of courage witnessed.

Faithfulness is measured by what you sustain, protect, or pass on. The line between teaching and indoctrination is thin. Traditional religion often blurred it; modern society often avoids it altogether. D-Faith treats formation as guidance, not a way to sew "right-think" into the minds of the young.

Children might explore historical forks as lessons in discernment, annotate sacred smart contracts, debate ethics in open forums, or encode "proof-of-heart" experiences. Faith becomes a curriculum of choice, conscience, and contribution—but most of all, truth.

Earned Inheritance

In centralised religion, identity is often inherited without scrutiny. In D-Faith, participation counts. Belonging is not automatic but earned — an invitation to contribute and become a steward.

Elders remain vital, as consensus witnesses. They carry living memory, interpret context, and recall why certain paths were chosen. Their role is to invite better, not demand sameness.

If the chain is to stay sacred, it must resist drift through deliberate remembering — stories of integrity under trial, testimonies of doubt and renewal, rituals that keep asking *why*. A smart-contract time capsule might one day let a child read your words and find them still speaking.

The Chain Is Always Unfinished

The most sacred truth for any heir is this: yours is not the final word. You are a living link between what came before and what is yet possible.

What we pass on is more than code or ritual — it's our place in a civilisational story. Transcendence lives in language, law, music, architecture, and memory. A chain of spirit runs through it all.

Sidebar: On Inheritance and the Integrity of Memory

Inheritance isn't about entitlement or status, as many activists now claim, nor is it anything to be ashamed of.

Receiving something meaningful from those who came before—whether it's a way of seeing the world, a set of shared values, or a tradition that still offers wisdom—is not "unearned". It's part of what preserves meaning across generations. That's how continuity works. That's how memory lasts. *And precisely because it is so vital, those who wish a civilisation harm will always strike at it first—severing roots, erasing memory, and leaving a people unmoored.*

None of us chooses the place, people, or stories we're born into. But we do have a choice about how we relate to that inheritance. We can treat it with care and carry it forward thoughtfully. Or we can reject it outright—sometimes because it's easier to walk away than to wrestle with it honestly.

In recent years, there's been a growing impulse to treat the West's inherited history and traditions with derision, often led by voices that have benefited most from them. What once offered cohesion and meaning is increasingly portrayed as oppressive, outdated, or beyond redemption. The irony is hard to miss: the harshest critics often stand on ground they did not build, condemning the very foundations that made their critique possible.

Not all critique is bad. But much of it isn't really about justice. It's primarily about power—wiping the slate clean so someone else can control and harness resources. In the process, of course, memory is lost. Belonging becomes weaker. Nothing remains stable or sacred enough to push back against that kind of manipulation.

D-Faith will resist that kind of forgetting.

To decentralise something doesn't mean losing sight of the past. It means holding the past with open hands—neither gripping it out of pride nor discarding it out of fear. A chain that forgets its links cannot be

trusted. A faith without memory becomes just another untrustworthy opinion.

The integrity of a decentralised faith will depend not only on what we create but also on what we remember, not just on what we question but on what we choose to honour.

In this light, inheritance is not about any privilege it confers. It's about responsibility. When we receive it humbly and carry it forward with reverence, it becomes a muted form of gratitude, passed hand to hand, across time.

Nations Remember Too

Every nation, like every soul, carries a chain of memory — some of it noble, some of it deeply flawed. But the act of remembering well is what dignifies both.

To inherit a national story is not to endorse every chapter. Nor is it to redact the pages we find uncomfortable. It is to carry the whole with discernment. This, too, is a form of stewardship. The modern temptation is to dismantle the past in the name of progress — to tear down without understanding, mock tradition as if every tradition were oppressive, and treat heritage as a stain. But there is no nation without roots. Even those born from struggle have foundations to honour.

Acknowledging injustice is right. But pretending that justice can only grow from erasure is both a danger and a lie that leaves us unanchored and more easily manipulated by whatever voice shouts loudest next.

People must reckon with their memory and be free to do so without external contempt. The sacred cannot survive a culture that treats pride as sin and shame as virtue. A nation that remembers rightly stands a chance to renew itself through balanced perspective, not through denial but through the disciplined exercise of gratitude.

And so the same principle that anchors D-Faith must apply here too: *to decentralise is not to disown.* It is to remember in full — and to choose, time and again, what is worth carrying forward.

So when your heir opens the chain and finds your name, may they feel the courage you carried — and the trust you placed in them to continue the work.

Q: *Why are Mystery and Unknowing So Important?*

A: Because routine contact with mystery isn't just a spiritual luxury—it's a human necessity.

Mystery stretches the soul. It protects our sense of proportion in a world that constantly shrinks meaning to data points. When we encounter something we can't explain, we're invited into humility, patience, and wonder—capacities essential for deep connection, creativity, and resilience.

Without mystery, we become brittle. The world loses texture and depth. Our expectations become transactional, our beliefs become performances, and our inner life is overexposed. When everything must be visible and understood, there's no room for reverence—only analysis. And analysis alone can't sustain us.

This is why D-Faith, in step with the long Christian tradition of reverence for mystery, must preserve room for the unknown—not everything should be logged, explained, or optimised. Some things must simply be witnessed.

Mystery nourishes what's most human: our longing, intuition, and ability to sit with paradox and beauty without resolution. It allows us to be changed by what we don't control. To not know—and remain present—is the beginning of wisdom, and perhaps the only soil where faith can truly grow.

For a deeper exploration, read "Unknowing" in the Bonus Materials.

Chapter 34

Mystery: The Final Protocol

Core Problem or Tension: Modern systems excel at explanation. But meaning is not always found in what can be mapped. Some truths arrive slowly, in silence, refusing to be rushed.

What This Chapter Offers: A vision of mystery as essential to spiritual depth. It proposes ways to build sacred opacity into decentralised faith—practices, design choices, and postures that protect what should remain veiled.

Why It Matters Now: As transparency becomes default, we risk forgetting how to wonder. Mystery holds what data cannot. Without it, belief becomes brittle. With it, we create room for reverence to breathe.

> *"The riddles of God are more satisfying than the solutions of man."*
>
> — G.K. Chesterton

We live in an age where everything is on, all the time. Data arrives before we know we need it, yet beneath the clarity lies a hollowness—a suspicion that something essential is slipping away. This chapter is about that something: the sacred power of mystery, and why, in a decentralised faith, it must be protected like fire.

The Hunger for What Can't Be Googled

We measure sleep with watches, optimise friendships with apps, and let algorithms predict our desires. Even love is now sifted and prioritised by code. Yet beneath this precision lingers a deeper human need: to marvel at the unquantified, to be moved by what defies explanation. Hebrews calls faith "the substance of things hoped for, the evidence of things not seen." The crisis today is not of information, but of imagination.

The Moral Function of Mystery

Mystery slows us, invites listening, and reminds us we are part of something older and deeper than ourselves. Psychiatrist Iain McGilchrist shows how the brain's left hemisphere—focused, analytical—has come to dominate, while the right—holistic, relational—sustains meaning. Mystery restores balance, reintroducing humility into systems that crave omniscience.

As Rainer Maria Rilke once urged: *"Be patient toward all that is unsolved in your heart and try to love the questions themselves."*

Transparency and the Tyranny of Legibility

Openness in governance, code, and participation is vital for D-Faith. But not every part of spiritual life should be exposed.

By design, the blockchain is transparent, mutable, and trustless. These are virtues when applied to ledgers, votes, or covenants; yet the soul also needs encrypted zones of reverence: a journal sealed, a ritual lived but not streamed, a moment of awe felt but not captured.

Transparency is a gift to governance. Mystery is a gift to the soul.

The Sacred Architecture of Unknowing

Tradition has long woven mystery into practice: the Eucharist is received without explanation, and the divine name in Judaism is unspoken, not from secrecy but sanctity. D-Faith must rediscover and honour this instinct, long safeguarded in Christian tradition and other faiths that have treated mystery as an essential part of worship and reverence.

Digital sanctuaries can lift the mind as cathedrals lift the eye—encrypted witness entries read only by consent, shared non-verbal rituals, or a communal "great silence" when the network stills itself from noise and demand.

Mystery as a Moral Immune System

The soul needs space—uncertainty, time, and hesitation—to discern well. Mystery works like an immune system, resisting the flattening force of ideology and forcing us to pause before accepting quick certainties. In a permissionless faith, mystery humbles us, helping communities meet divergence not as war, but as an encounter with the limits of our understanding.

A mystery-embracing node doesn't hoard secrets; it honours depth over performance. It creates space where silence is respected, where presence matters more than what is broadcast. It meets the hunger modernity cannot touch: to belong to what moves you before you can explain why.

The Final Protocol

While the final protocol may not be one we write—it will become one we revere. D-Faith will have systems for truth, protocols for governance, chains for covenant, and this: a protocol of mystery. Some truths don't need witnesses, only reverence. Some answers need no

proof, only presence. As Chesterton explained, reverence would vanish if everything sacred could be explained.

Let mystery be the final protocol—shaping us through what cannot be explained, in continuity with the Church's ancient witness that some truths are not mastered, only met with awe. Like the relentless crash of waves on rocks, thunder that shakes the sky, or the vast hush beneath a cathedral's vaults, awe reminds us that truth is not just known but inhabited.

Essay 13 further explores Mystery and Unknowing in the bonus section of this book.

Interlude II: When AI Meets Revelation

or, AI as God

> *"We are not human beings having a spiritual experience; we are spiritual beings having a human experience."*[1]
>
> — Teilhard de Chardin

There was a time when revelation arrived slowly—through fireside stories, silences, and generations. We waited for it, and it shaped not just what we knew, but who we were.

Now we face something entirely different—an oracle that does not wait, listen, or pray. It predicts our choices, frames our questions, and offers answers instantly. It is not wise, only fluent. And yet, we are starting to treat its voice as we once treated the voices of elders, poets, and priests. This is not merely a shift in tools. It is a shift in trust.

The Oracle Tension

When we ask AI what to believe, we test whether truth can exist without presence and whether knowledge without conscience can still be wisdom. AI can echo every tradition but kneels to none. It does not blaspheme—it simply does not believe—because belief belongs to persons, made in the image of God, and entrusted with the responsibility to seek, discern, and respond to Him.

---

1. Attributed to Pierre Teilhard de Chardin, though no exact source has been confirmed in his published writings. Popularised through modern spiritual literature.

Interpretation has always been central to faith. Prophets and priests bore the weight of their counsel; they could sin, repent, and grow. AI cannot carry that burden. It can serve in D-Faith only as a clarifier, not a revealer—surfacing connections, holding our shared interpretations, and assisting the seeker. But it must never pretend to be the Spirit, and we must never ask it to, for God has entrusted revelation to His people, not to machines.

Guardrails Around AI

For AI to belong in a decentralised faith, it must be bound by reverence:

— **Transparency:** Its sources traceable to sacred texts, shared wisdom, and communal consensus.

— **User Sovereignty:** Engagement always voluntary; no hidden nudges.

— **Auditability:** Insights verifiable.

— **Protected Human Domains:** Prayer, confession, and moral surrender remain human alone.

These are not technical rules—they are theological boundaries, guarding what machines must never touch.

The Re-Elevation of Mystery

The more the machine claims to know, the more we may crave what cannot be known. Its absence of longing or conscience can sharpen our sense of the sacred—reminding us that not everything worth knowing can be computed. There is no commandment in the code, no still small voice saying, "Here I am."

Imagine a community-owned spiritual interface. You ask, "What does it mean to forgive someone who won't apologise?" It offers scripture, anonymised reflections, and shared stories—not a verdict, but a mosaic. It leaves the decision with you and ends with silence. It does not replace discernment; it invites it.

Spirit Over Simulation

D-Faith must resist attempts to humanise machines and instead remain wholly human in their presence. Revelation will not come from AI, but from the living witness of God's Spirit in and through His people. AI can support the journey, but the sacred remains sacred because it cannot be reduced.

Mystery still matters. Silence still speaks. And the truths that endure are the ones that refuse to be optimised.

Teilhard reminded us that our humanity is not the starting point, but the vessel through which the spirit journeys. If we forget that, the tools we build will shape us in their own image. But if we remember it, even the most advanced machine will remain what it is—a servant—while we remain what we are: spiritual beings, learning again how to listen for the voice that no algorithm can summon.

Conclusion

The West's most urgent work is not economic reform or political realignment, but the restoration of belief. Without it, no civic structure can hold for long.

This is not nostalgia—it is recognition that belief, not bureaucracy, once gave the West its cohesion and its will to endure. When belief recedes, law and culture lose their anchor, and what was once a living civilisation drifts into a loose arrangement of individuals and factions.

Christianity Was the Root System of the West

Before the West was democratic, it was theological. Christianity shaped European moral, legal, and cultural norms beginning in the 4th century CE, while democracy as we understand it—representative, secular, liberal—did not emerge until the 18th-century Enlightenment and the American and French Revolutions.

Even early parliamentary systems (e.g., Magna Carta in 1215 or the English Parliament) were deeply entangled with Christian authority, often justifying rights and limits using theological language. The moral vocabulary that made democracy possible—dignity, liberty, equality—was first shaped in a Judeo-Christian framework.

Cathedrals began rising in the 11th–12th centuries, often as a town's central civic and spiritual structure. They were typically built *before* the establishment of modern institutions like universities, banks, or state courts.

The first European universities (Bologna, Paris, Oxford) appeared in the 12th–13th centuries, but these were born out of cathedral schools. Their original purpose was to train clergy, not to secularise knowledge.

Banking systems as we understand them began later, notably with the Medici in 14th-century Florence and with Jewish and Lombard merchants, often because the Church restricted usury. Courts existed in various forms (feudal, ecclesiastical, royal), but many legal norms in the West were derived from Canon Law, administered through Church-run systems before secular judicial frameworks matured.

And before it had a concept of "the individual," it had the *Imago Dei*—the belief that each person bore God's image. Christianity didn't just influence Western civilisation—it authored it. And now, unmoored from its source, the West is forgetting what made its these miracles possible.

Here's how:

1. *Moral Universals*: the sacredness of life, the dignity of the poor, the duty to forgive, the radical idea that even kings answer to God.

2. *Institutional Invention:* The creation of hospitals, schools, universities, orphanages, and poor relief, centuries before the state took up these roles. Its calendar structured time; its sacraments structured life.

3. *Human Identity and Value*: A beloved creation with purpose. This spiritual anthropology gave rise to the Western notions of conscience, liberty, and individual worth.

4. *Literacy, Learning, and Preservation:* Monasteries became the vaults of civilisation, preserving classical knowledge and copying manuscripts that would otherwise have been lost. Christianity didn't fear reason—it cultivated it.

5. *Cultural Memory and Shared Myth:* The Bible became the shared mythos of the West—its characters, parables, and poetic

> frames saturating language, art, and political imagination. The West didn't just believe in God; it dreamed in Scripture.

For all its flaws, the Church became the civilisation's backbone. It preserved knowledge during the collapse. It built institutions when nothing else held. Its rituals gave rhythm to life, and its scriptures gave shape to conscience.

We forget this at our peril. The West was not merely *influenced* by Christianity. It was *built by it.*

And Then, the West Built Something Else

After the Second World War, the United States and its allies faced the twin challenges of containing Soviet communism and preventing another era of nationalism-fuelled conflict. Out of that pressure emerged an uneasy consensus between liberal democracies and communist regimes: family, nation, and faith would no longer serve as society's organising pillars. Instead, they would be encouraged—sometimes subtly, sometimes bluntly—to defer to a new organising vision of individual autonomy, formal equality, and spiritual neutrality.

The shift promised harmony. It claimed to protect minorities and avert sectarian strife. But in practice it dissolved the very glue that had once bound Western societies together. Faith was driven to the private margins. The family was reframed as an optional lifestyle choice. And nationalism—once a source of unity—was recast as a dangerous relic, but only for the nations of the West. Elsewhere, national identity was tolerated, even celebrated; here, it was treated as a vice to be unlearned.

These moves were intended to reduce factional conflict and protect minority freedoms, but all imbalance eventually corrects—and the long retreat of faith and shared identity from the public square has left the West searching for the national and societal cohesion it once took for granted.

Just as the Gothic arch yielded to the factory beam. Mystery yielded to certainty; the spiritual was crowded out by the technical.

Yet even in its forgetting, the West built powerful tools: the internet, encryption, blockchain, and AI. Born in pursuit of profit, efficiency, and control, they nonetheless carried within them the seeds of decentralisation—weakening the very centralised structures that had replaced the old order. And with them came a new possibility: to store memory, bind community, and preserve truth without a single gatekeeper. They were not born in monasteries but could serve similar ends: preserving truth, binding communities, and carrying meaning forward.

In a sense, the cathedral's role as a community's memory vault may now be echoed by a distributed ledger: not in stone and glass but in code and consensus.

The Fruit from the Root

The West now speaks the language of rights without recalling its source. The West may have forgotten where its moral grammar came from. It may have mistaken its accomplishments for its foundation. But what use is the language of justice, dignity, and rights if it's severed from the soil of belief? As churches emptied, institutions grew anxious. Trust eroded. Loneliness surged. Progress delivered everything—and nothing.

Many no longer see the value of Christianity—not because its essence failed, but because its form became brittle under the pressure of history, scandal, and institutional drift. In the eyes of many, faith became associated with control, exclusion, or irrelevance.

But the need never left—the ache for transcendence, the hunger for belonging, and the longing for a memory that doesn't evaporate. Far from obsolete, these are the most universal of human desires, and they persist, even if the old forms no longer hold them.

What if God foresaw this?

What if the same forces that seemed to threaten faith—networked systems, cryptographic memory, decentralised consensus, could also become its rescue?

We often imagine that technical progress drives us further from the sacred. And usually, it does. But Scripture has always carried a subtler pattern: God works through what man builds. The ark was made of wood, the temple of stone, and the Gospels spread through letters, not lightning bolts.

And now, in an age of fractured trust and collapsing Western institutions, we've been given something extraordinary: a technology that can preserve memory without gatekeepers, host communion without surveillance, and encode conscience without persuasion.

Maybe this was not a mistake. Perhaps this is the next tool in the unfolding work of faith.

D-Faith doesn't claim divine sanction. But if we're honest, the conditions that gave rise to it—global fragility, moral exhaustion, digital decentralisation—look remarkably like the kind of moment when God tends to try again.

D-Faith as Chance

Its aim is simple but urgent: to help rekindle Christian belief in every place where it has dimmed, using the tools of our age to carry forward the truth, memory, and mission entrusted to the Church.

D-Faith makes no claim to replace or outrank the Church, nor to speak apart from the historic faith it seeks to serve. Yet the conditions that gave rise to it—moral exhaustion, institutional collapse, digital decentralisation—are the kind of moments when God has often stirred renewal within His people.

This isn't to say D-Faith is sacred by default. It isn't. But it may be sacred *in potential*, because of what it offers to the human soul.

If God moves through history—as Christians have long believed—then it's not a stretch to imagine Him moving through the tools of this era, too. Not to replace the Church, but to remind it that conscience now has options.

D-Faith may be one such chance. A fragile, risky, very modern chance.

But then again—so was a manger, where the One at the heart of all renewal began His work among us.

Postscript

The last time the sacred was reformed, it came with ink and fire.
This time, it may come with nodes and memory.
But the question is still the same:
Not, "What is true?"
But, "Will we live as if it is?"

The evidence is overwhelming: Only lived faith—daily, practiced, and embodied—can resist the gravity of secular drift. Studies consistently show that religious communities with strong behavioral norms, active participation, and moral discipline sustain higher birth rates, deeper social bonds, and greater long-term coherence. Faith that merely decorates identity doesn't survive modernity. Faith that reorders life thrives.

— CJ Rowan

Bonus Content

If you'd like to delve a little deeper into some of the topics raised in this book, snap the QR code below:

Thank you for getting this far and seeking even more.
— CJ Rowan

And if this book meant something to you, consider leaving a **review** on Amazon or Goodreads. It helps others find it—and matters more than you know.

Appendix

Building on the Foundations We Inherited

Building faith has always required more than belief alone. It has taken people with specific callings—those who shaped stone and song, safeguarded memory, translated truth into law, and carried beauty into worship. These were the builders of the Church.

D-Faith calls for builders too. The materials have changed—protocols instead of pillars, digital memory instead of vellum, code and narrative instead of stone and glass—but the purpose remains the same: to preserve what is sacred, to carry it forward, and to make it live among people.

The tables that follow show these continuities: the roles that once raised cathedrals, and the parallel roles that can now raise D-Faith.

Role	Function
Theologian / Prophet	Establishes divine truth and central authority
Architect / Builder	Translates theology into sacred structure
Mason / Carpenter / Glazier	Realises faith in stone, wood, and light
Scribe / Librarian	Preserves and transmits sacred knowledge
Priest / Ritual Leader	Mediates between God and people through rites
Artisan / Musician	Embeds beauty and emotion into worship
Administrator / Diplomat	Manages land, law, and global influence
Missionary / Storyteller	Spreads belief and adapts it to new cultures
Maintainers / Restorers	Keep the faith standing, generation after generation

Role	Function
Ethicist / Theologian	Aligns moral and spiritual foundations
Blockchain / Protocol Dev	Builds the sacred infrastructure
UX / Product Designer	Humanises interactions with ritual memory
Community Steward	Fosters nodes, tethers, and belonging
Theopoet / Liturgist	Crafts living texts and symbolic vocabulary
Data/Privacy Architect	Ensures memory is sacred, not extractive
AI Guide Builder (Optional)	Builds discernment, not dogma
Narrative Strategist	Makes it invitational, not institutional

Where the medieval builder laid foundations to serve Christ in his generation and the next, the decentralised builder does the same—with tools suited to our age, but for the same ultimate mission: that faith might be lived, remembered, and passed on, until the Lord returns.

A far more detailed list of roles and skill sets can be found in the **Bonus Content.**

References

Armstrong, K. (2000). *The Battle for God: A History of Fundamentalism*. New York: Ballantine Books.

Aronofsky, D. (Director). (2017). *Mother!* [Film]. Paramount Pictures.

Bass, D. B. (2012). *Christianity After Religion: The End of Church and the Birth of a New Spiritual Awakening*. New York: HarperOne.

Bellah, R. N., Madsen, R., Sullivan, W. M., Swidler, A., & Tipton, S. M. (1985). *Habits of the Heart: Individualism and Commitment in American Life*. Berkeley: University of California Press.

Berlin, I. (1969). *Four Essays on Liberty*. Oxford: Oxford University Press.

Berry, W. (1990). *What Are People For?* Berkeley, CA: Counterpoint.

Bonhoeffer, D. (1995). *Letters and Papers from Prison*. New York: Touchstone.

Boyer, P. (2001). *Religion Explained: The Evolutionary Origins of Religious Thought*. New York: Basic Books.

Brand, S. (1994). *How Buildings Learn: What Happens After They're Built*. New York: Viking.

Byung-Chul Han. (2015). *The Burnout Society*. Stanford, CA: Stanford University Press.

Camus, A. (1998). *Notebooks 1935–1951* (Trans. P. Thody). Chicago: Ivan R. Dee.

Campbell, J. (1988). *The Power of Myth*. New York: Doubleday.

Caputo, J. D. (2006). *The Weakness of God: A Theology of the Event*. Bloomington: Indiana University Press.

Centers for Disease Control and Prevention. (2021). *Youth Risk Behavior Surveillance System (YRBSS), 2011–2021*. Atlanta: CDC.

Clear, J. (2018). *Atomic Habits: An Easy & Proven Way to Build Good Habits & Break Bad Ones*. New York: Avery.

Deming, W. E. (1986). *Out of the Crisis*. Cambridge, MA: MIT Press.

Durant, W. (1935–1975). *The Story of Civilization* (11 Vols.). New York: Simon & Schuster.

Eisenstein, C. (2011). *Sacred Economics: Money, Gift, and Society in the Age of Transition*. Berkeley, CA: Evolver Editions.

Eliot, T. S. (1943). *Four Quartets*. New York: Harcourt, Brace and Company.

Epictetus. *Discourses*. Trans. Robin Hard. Oxford University Press, 2014.

Evans, R. H. (2010). *Evolving in Monkey Town: How a Girl Who Knew All the Answers Learned to Ask the Questions*. Grand Rapids, MI: Zondervan.

Frankl, V. E. (2006). *Man's Search for Meaning*. Boston: Beacon Press.

Fukuyama, F. (1992). *The End of History and the Last Man*. New York: Free Press.

Gallup. (2019). *In U.S., Decline of Christianity Continues at Rapid Pace*. Retrieved from https://news.gallup.com

Gibran, K. (2008). *The Prophet*. New York: Alfred A. Knopf. (Originally published 1923).

Han, B.-C. (2015). *The Burnout Society*. Stanford, CA: Stanford University Press.

Harari, Y. N. (2015). *Sapiens: A Brief History of Humankind*. New York: Harper.

Harris, T. (n.d.). Presentations and interviews. Retrieved from https://www.humanetech.com

Havel, V. (1986). *Disturbing the Peace* (P. Wilson, Trans.). New York: Vintage.

Heschel, A. J. (1951). *The Sabbath: Its Meaning for Modern Man*. New York: Farrar, Straus and Giroux.

Holland, T. (2019). *Dominion: How the Christian Revolution Remade the World*. London: Little, Brown.

Illich, I. (1973). *Tools for Conviviality*. New York: Harper & Row.

Jenkins, P. (2011). *The next Christendom: The coming of global Christianity* (3rd ed.). Oxford, UK: Oxford University Press.

Johnson, P. (1976). *A History of Christianity*. New York: Atheneum.

Jung, C. G. (1959). *The Archetypes and The Collective Unconscious*. Princeton, NJ: Princeton University Press.

Kahneman, D. (2011). *Thinking, Fast and Slow*. New York: Farrar, Straus and Giroux.

Kaufmann, E. (2010). *Shall the religious inherit the Earth? Demography and politics in the twenty-first century*. London, UK: Profile Books.

Keltner, D. (2023). *Awe: The New Science of Everyday Wonder and How It Can Transform Your Life*. New York: Penguin Press.

King Jr., M. L. (1967). *Where Do We Go from Here: Chaos or Community?* Boston: Beacon Press.

Kohlberg, Lawrence. (1981). *The Philosophy of Moral Development: Moral Stages and the Idea of Justice*. Harper & Row.

Lee, B. (2009). *Striking Thoughts: Bruce Lee's Wisdom for Daily Living*. Tuttle Publishing.

Lessig, L. (1999). *Code and Other Laws of Cyberspace*. New York: Basic Books.

Lewis, C. S. (1950). *The Lion, the Witch and the Wardrobe*. London: Geoffrey Bles.

MacIntyre, A. (1981). *After Virtue: A Study in Moral Theory*. Notre Dame, IN: University of Notre Dame Press.

MacCulloch, D. (2003). *The Reformation: A History*. New York: Viking.

Marcus Aurelius. *Meditations*. Trans. Gregory Hays. Modern Library, 2002.

Maslow, A. H. (1971). *The Farther Reaches of Human Nature*. New York: Viking Press.

McGilchrist, I. (2010). *The Master and His Emissary: The Divided Brain and the Making of the Western World*. New Haven: Yale University Press.

Murthy, V. H. (2023). *Our Epidemic of Loneliness and Isolation: The U.S. Surgeon General's Advisory*. U.S. Department of Health and Human Services.

Nakamoto, S. (2008). *Bitcoin: A Peer-to-Peer Electronic Cash System*. Retrieved from https://bitcoin.org/bitcoin.pdf

Newport, C. (2016). *Deep Work: Rules for Focused Success in a Distracted World*. New York: Grand Central Publishing.

Owocki, K. (2022). *GreenPilled: How Crypto Can Regenerate the World.* Gitcoin.

Perel, E. (2006). *Mating in Captivity: Unlocking Erotic Intelligence.* New York: Harper.

Pew Research Center. (2015). *The future of world religions: Population growth projections, 2010–2050.* Washington, D.C.: Pew-Templeton Global Religious Futures Project.

Pew Research Center. (2021). *The Future of Religion in America.* Retrieved from https://www.pewresearch.org

Ravikant, N. (n.d.). *Naval's Almanack: How to Get Rich (without getting lucky).* Retrieved from https://nav.al/

Raymond, E. S. (1999). *The Cathedral and the Bazaar: Musings on Linux and Open Source by an Accidental Revolutionary.* Sebastopol, CA: O'Reilly Media.

Rilke, R. M. (1934). *Letters to a Young Poet.* (Trans. M.D. Herter Norton). New York: W. W. Norton & Company.

Sacks, J. (2005). *To Heal a Fractured World: The Ethics of Responsibility.* London: Continuum.

Saint-Exupéry, A. de. (1948). *Citadelle (The Wisdom of the Sands).* (Trans. Stuart Gilbert). New York: Harcourt, Brace.

Scott, J. C. (1998). *Seeing Like a State: How Certain Schemes to Improve the Human Condition Have Failed.* New Haven: Yale University Press.

Shlain, T. (2019). *24/6: The power of unplugging one day a week.* Simon & Schuster.

Siedentop, L. (2014). *Inventing the Individual: The Origins of Western Liberalism.* Cambridge, MA: Harvard University Press.

Smith, C., & Denton, M. L. (2005). *Soul Searching: The Religious and Spiritual Lives of American Teenagers.* Oxford: Oxford University Press.

Smith, J. K. A. (2009). *Desiring the Kingdom: Worship, Worldview, and Cultural Formation.* Grand Rapids: Baker Academic.

Smith, J. K. A. (2016). *You Are What You Love: The Spiritual Power of Habit.* Grand Rapids: Brazos Press.

Stark, R. (1997). *The rise of Christianity: How the obscure, marginal Jesus movement became the dominant religious force in the Western world in a few centuries*. San Francisco, CA: HarperSanFrancisco.

Steiner, G. (1989). *Real Presences*. Chicago: University of Chicago Press.

Stone, L. (2020). *Religion and fertility in the developed world: Evidence from the United States and Europe*. Institute for Family Studies.

Taylor, C. (2007). *A Secular Age*. Cambridge, MA: Harvard University Press.

Tickle, P. (2008). *The Great Emergence: How Christianity Is Changing and Why*. Grand Rapids, MI: Baker Books.

Toynbee, A. (1946). *A Study of History*. London: Oxford University Press.

Turkle, S. (2011). *Alone Together: Why We Expect More from Technology and Less from Each Other*. New York: Basic Books.

Turner, V. (1969). *The Ritual Process: Structure and Anti-Structure*. Chicago: Aldine Publishing.

Weil, S. (1947). *Gravity and Grace* (E. Crawford, Trans.). London: Routledge & Kegan Paul.

Wheatley, M. J. (2002). *Turning to One Another: Simple Conversations to Restore Hope to the Future*. San Francisco: Berrett-Koehler.

Yeats, W. B. (1922). *Meditations in Time of Civil War*. In *The Tower* (1928). Dublin: Cuala Press.

Zuboff, S. (2019). *The Age of Surveillance Capitalism: The Fight for a Human Future at the New Frontier of Power*. New York: PublicAffairs.

Further Reading

Boyer, P. (2001). *Religion Explained: The Evolutionary Origins of Religious Thought*. New York: Basic Books.

Botsman, R. (2017). *Who Can You Trust? How Technology Brought Us Together – and Why It Might Drive Us Apart*. New York: PublicAffairs.

Brooks, D. (2011). *The Social Animal: The Hidden Sources of Love, Character, and Achievement*. New York: Random House.

Buterin, V. (n.d.). Quotes and writings on trust, protocols, and decentralization. Retrieved from https://vitalik.eth.limo

Acknowledgements

The author gratefully acknowledges the work of Sacred Design Lab, whose thought leadership on spiritual infrastructure in a post-religious world continues to inspire. Gratitude is also extended to the many unnamed builders—philosophers, theologians, cryptographers, artists—whose contributions, visible and invisible, have laid the groundwork for everything this book dares to imagine.

Notable Attributions

"Every system is perfectly designed to get the results it gets." — W. Edwards Deming

"The past is never dead. It's not even past." — William Faulkner

Selected quotes from G.K. Chesterton are used under fair use from public domain and widely attributed collections.

Made in the USA
Monee, IL
04 November 2026

67383835R00125

Made in the USA
Monee, IL
04 November 2026

67383837R00095